Table of contents

Introduction

Welcome to Dental School: Why This Path Matters

Congratulations on choosing to embark on one of the most challenging and rewarding journeys out there: dental school! This isn't just any academic pursuit; it's a commitment to learning the art and science of improving lives through oral health. Dental school isn't only about acquiring medical knowledge—it's also about developing skills and habits that will shape your entire career. Through these pages, you'll find guidance on study strategies, tips for overcoming procrastination, insights into self-discipline, and even hygiene tips that will make your journey smoother. Along the way, you'll also hear personal stories from students who have walked this path before, so you know you're not alone in facing the hurdles ahead.

Why Choose Dentistry?

For many of us, the road to dentistry isn't a straightforward one. Maybe it was a fascination with biology and anatomy that drew you in, or perhaps it was an admiration for the dentist who made a lasting impact on your life. Dentistry is unique in its blend of precision, care, and artistry. You're not just fixing teeth—you're helping people regain confidence, alleviate pain, and improve their overall well-being. And though the journey may feel daunting at times, that purpose—of truly helping others—becomes a powerful motivator on the toughest days.

Some choose dentistry because it's one of the few fields where they can both use their hands and engage their minds every day. It's a career that demands focus and skill, yet allows for creativity. You'll become adept at using fine motor skills and meticulous techniques to create something beautiful and functional. And in the end, you're not just changing smiles—you're changing lives. There's an old saying, "A smile is the universal welcome," and in dentistry, you have the privilege of making that welcome possible for so many.

The Reality: A Path Filled with Challenges

But let's be real: dental school is no walk in the park. There's an intensity to the learning process that can feel overwhelming. You'll face long hours of lectures and labs, endless exams, and practice sessions that require you to perfect techniques down to the millimetre. There's a pressure that comes with knowing the impact your work will have on a real person's health and comfort, and this expectation of precision can be daunting. A small error on a test can mean a simple mistake, but a small slip during a procedure could mean a patient's discomfort.

Many dental students have stories of their first shaky moments in lab, hands trembling as they attempted their first cavity filling on a practice mannequin. "The difference between a filling and a failure is in a few millimeters," an instructor might remind you, and they're right. But this level of precision isn't just a hurdle—it's also a skill that builds your resilience. As you practice and progress, you'll start to feel the rewards of honing these skills. With every small success, you're reminded that you're working toward something bigger than yourself.

The Rewards: More Than Just a Degree

With all these challenges come unparalleled rewards. Dentistry offers a unique sense of accomplishment, one that's as personal as it is professional. Imagine the day you treat your first patient. It's a blend of pride, nervousness, and excitement as you realize that the skills you've spent years developing will genuinely impact someone's life. Over time, as you gain confidence, you'll also feel a growing pride in your craft. You'll know that with every patient you help, you're making a difference.

Beyond the clinic, dental school creates a community of like-minded individuals. Your classmates are on this journey with you, facing the same sleepless nights, exam pressures, and practical challenges. They'll become study partners, allies, and close friends—people who understand the highs and lows that come with this field. Together, you'll share frustrations, celebrate each small victory, and ultimately, grow into skilled professionals side by side.

This book is here to be your companion through the ups and downs of dental school, offering you practical tips, motivation, and personal reflections. Whether it's learning study techniques, managing your time, or navigating those daunting lab days, these pages are designed to support you. Through real stories and insights, you'll see that others have faced these same obstacles and come out stronger. There's an African proverb that says, "Smooth seas do not make skillful sailors," and the same is true in dental school—the challenges will shape you into a stronger, more capable dentist.

As you embark on this rigorous yet fulfilling path, remember that you're not alone. Every late night, every small victory, and every new skill mastered brings you one step closer to becoming the dentist you aspire to be. This journey will test your resolve, but it will also shape you in ways you can't yet imagine. So, take a deep breath, lean into the challenges, and trust that you're on the right path. You're here because you have something to offer—a gift for helping others, one smile at a time.

Purpose of the Book: Your Guide Through Dental School

This book was created with a clear mission: to equip you, as a dental student, with practical strategies for academic success, well-being, and personal growth throughout your studies. Dental school is demanding, and success requires more than just intelligence; it takes effective study habits, strong self-discipline, and a commitment to personal care. This guide will walk with you through those challenges, offering strategies to manage the unique workload, maintain balance, and thrive—academically and personally.

But this book isn't just another dry study manual. What makes it different is its blend of AI-assisted insight and genuine human experiences from those who have been exactly where you are now. It's an authentic guide to navigating the highs and lows of dental school, combining practical advice with real stories and lessons from past students who know the struggles, successes, and everything in between. From handling the pressures of exam week to finding moments of joy in the journey, this book is designed to be a companion and a support system.

Think of this book as a trusted friend, a mentor, and a guide all in one. It's filled with real-world tips and lessons we all wish we'd known in our first years of dental school. You'll find strategies for efficient studying, managing stress, and cultivating self-discipline, all while keeping your personal health in check. The journey won't be easy—dental school will test your patience, focus, and resilience—but with the right tools and a positive outlook, you can embrace each part of it.

In the pages ahead, you'll find techniques to help you manage your time, overcome procrastination, and stay organized during those late nights when assignments and practicals start piling up. You'll also get a glimpse into the daily life of dental students, with anecdotes that bring these lessons to life.

As the African proverb says, "Wisdom is like a baobab tree; no one individual can embrace it." That's what this book offers—a collective well of wisdom that can guide you, support you, and even make you smile on the tougher days.

So, let's dive into this journey, face the challenges, celebrate the small victories, and make the most of these transformative years together. By the time you reach the end of this book—and dental school—you'll not only be ready to build a successful career, but you'll also have the strength and confidence to make a difference in the lives of others, one smile at a time.

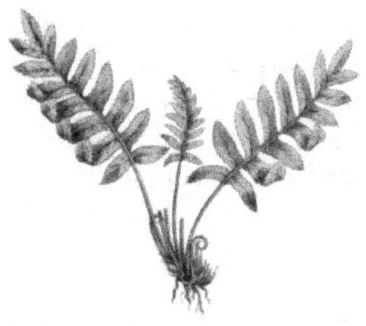

Turning Disappointment into Purpose

Embracing Dental School After Medical College Setbacks

For many who dream of a career in healthcare, medicine often seems like the ultimate goal—a golden ticket to a life of purpose and prestige. Yet, when that goal slips out of reach—whether due to tough competition, unforeseen circumstances, or simply a missed opportunity—it can feel profoundly disheartening. The path you'd envisioned is suddenly blocked, and the weight of disappointment can be heavy, leading to feelings of dejection that may linger longer than we'd like.

However, choosing to enter dental school after not securing a seat in medical college is not a consolation prize; it's a new journey filled with unique opportunities and rich rewards. It is said that "when one door closes, another opens," and this can be particularly true in the realm of healthcare. Dental school, while initially perceived as a second choice by some, offers a path that is just as impactful, rewarding, and essential to overall health as medicine itself.

I remember a classmate, Raj, who had always dreamed of being a doctor. He worked tirelessly, fuelled by passion and ambition, only to find himself facing the bitter disappointment of not gaining admission to medical school. For weeks, he wrestled with feelings of failure, struggling to see any value in what felt like a detour. However, in a moment of introspection, he decided to explore dental school instead. Raj discovered that dentistry was not only a way to work in healthcare but also an opportunity to build meaningful relationships with patients, relieve pain, and restore confidence. He realized that helping someone regain their smile was just as noble a calling as treating illnesses.

This shift in perspective is crucial. Dentistry may not have been the original dream, but it's a field that requires precision, skill, and artistry. I recall my own experience during the first week of dental school when I held a dental handpiece for the first time. My hands trembled as I practiced filling a cavity on a mannequin, the pressure of the moment weighing on me. Yet, in that small victory, I felt an exhilarating sense of accomplishment. It dawned on me that each small step was a building block toward mastering a craft that could profoundly impact lives.

In the words of Confucius, "Our greatest glory is not in never falling, but in rising every time we fall." This wisdom rings true in the lives of many dental students who, like Raj and myself, had to confront setbacks on their paths to success. The journey through dental school can be arduous, filled with long hours of study and practice, yet with each challenge comes the chance to grow and discover a new passion.

Ultimately, the opportunity to practice dentistry offers a way to fulfill a commitment to helping others, alleviating pain, and improving lives. It's a realization that many find in their first encounters with patients. For instance, Priya, another friend from dental school, had a transformative experience during a community outreach program. She helped a young woman suffering from severe dental pain, and the relief in the patient's eyes was immediate and heartwarming. In that moment, Priya understood that her role as a dentist could restore not just physical health but also a sense of self-worth and joy.

The decision to pivot from medicine to dentistry can be daunting, but it is essential to embrace the path you've chosen with confidence. It is about turning disappointment into an opportunity for growth and exploration. With every new skill learned and every patient helped, the initial sting of unmet expectations fades, revealing a journey filled with potential, purpose, and a profound ability to impact lives.

So remember: when one door closes, take the time to explore what lies beyond the next one. You may find that the path ahead is just as fulfilling and meaningful as the one you thought you had lost.

Acknowledge and Process the Disappointment

The journey of pursuing a career in healthcare often comes with its share of setbacks, and when those moments arise, it's essential to pause and allow yourself to feel the disappointment. The first step in overcoming any setback is acknowledging the feelings that come with it. There's a natural sense of loss when your dreams seem to slip away, especially after you've invested so much effort, time, and emotion into a singular goal. In these moments, it's important to remember the wise saying, "It's okay to not be okay." Feeling disappointed doesn't signify weakness; it's a testament to the passion you held for your aspirations.

I remember my friend Maya, who dreamed of becoming a physician since childhood. She worked tirelessly throughout her undergraduate years, often sacrificing social events and personal time for her studies. When the acceptance letters were sent out, Maya faced the harsh reality of not being among the chosen few. The weight of that disappointment felt unbearable at first. She spent days in reflection, grappling with the sense of loss that had settled over her like a thick fog.

However, Maya soon realized that processing her feelings was a crucial part of moving forward. Instead of burying her disappointment, she chose to embrace it. She began journaling her thoughts, pouring out her emotions onto the pages with honesty and vulnerability. Through writing, she found clarity, understanding that it was okay to grieve the dream she had long held. Her journal became a safe space for her feelings, a place where she could explore her disappointments without judgment.

In addition to journaling, Maya reached out to her family and friends, sharing her experiences and emotions. Talking to a trusted friend, who had faced a similar setback, allowed her to see that she wasn't alone. There's a proverb that says, "A shared burden is half a burden." By voicing her disappointment, Maya lightened her emotional load, gaining perspective and support from those who truly cared for her well-being.

In her search for healing, Maya also took up painting—a hobby she had once loved but had set aside during her intense study period. With each brushstroke, she began to rediscover not just her creativity, but also her passion for life beyond the confines of academia. Painting became a therapeutic outlet, allowing her to express her emotions in ways that words could not. It reminded her that while she faced a setback, her identity was not solely defined by her career ambitions.

Allowing yourself the grace to feel and process disappointment is a necessary step toward healing. It's essential to give yourself time to reflect, to honour the effort you put forth, and to embrace the emotions that arise. As Maya learned, the road to resilience begins with acknowledging your feelings and understanding that setbacks, while painful, can lead to unexpected growth and new opportunities. When faced with disappointment, remember that "Every cloud has a silver lining."

By leaning into your emotions and seeking constructive outlets, you can transform your setback into a stepping stone toward a fulfilling future.

Reframe the "Failure" as a Redirection

The next step in overcoming disappointment is to shift your perspective and reframe the experience. Failing to get into medical school doesn't mean you lack intelligence, dedication, or the potential to make a real difference. In truth, healthcare fields are incredibly competitive, and everyone's journey is unique. Not securing a spot in one program doesn't define your abilities, nor does it limit the impact you can have on others. There's a saying that "Every setback is a setup for a comeback," and for many, finding a new path can lead to unexpected fulfilment.

Dentistry, like medicine, combines science, artistry, and patient care. It's a highly respected profession that allows you to transform people's health, confidence, and overall quality of life. When you're working one-on-one with a patient, easing their pain or helping them feel comfortable with their smile again, you're making a profound difference. In this way, dentistry offers the same opportunity to heal and connect with others, reminding us that no single career path holds a monopoly on fulfilment or purpose.

Sometimes, what seems like failure is really the universe nudging us in a different direction. I recall my friend Raj, who had dreamed of becoming a doctor for as long as he could remember. Medicine was his goal, and he invested years of effort, energy, and sacrifice into that dream. But when the acceptance letters arrived, his wasn't among them. Disheartened, Raj spent weeks reflecting on what had happened, and for a while, he felt lost. Eventually, he decided to try dental school, thinking of it as a practical alternative.

At first, Raj's heart wasn't fully in it. But as he started his classes, something shifted. He discovered that he enjoyed the intricate, hands-on work dentistry required. With each lab and clinic session, he felt a new excitement as he realized that dentistry wasn't just an alternative; it was an opportunity to fulfill his healthcare aspirations in a meaningful, tangible way. Raj began to see his new path not as a consolation prize but as a redirection—an opportunity to make a profound impact on his patients' lives, just as he had always hoped.

This reframing helped Raj let go of the notion that dentistry was a "second choice" and embrace it as a fulfilling, impactful career on its own. Like the proverb says, "When life gives you lemons, make lemonade." By shifting his perspective, Raj found a way to use his initial setback as a stepping stone toward a new and satisfying career.

Dentistry, with its blend of science, skill, and direct patient interaction, offers its own unique rewards. It's not about settling; it's about staying open to possibilities and seeing beyond a single definition of success. For many, the journey into dentistry after not securing a medical seat becomes a turning point. They come to find that while their path didn't look exactly like they'd imagined, it was just as valuable—and perhaps even more fulfilling than they'd expected.

Find New Inspiration in Dentistry

See Dentistry as a Field of Endless Growth and Opportunity

When you first imagined a career in healthcare, what drew you in? Was it a desire to help others, a fascination with human anatomy, or perhaps a dream of making a meaningful impact on people's lives? While medicine might have been your initial goal, dentistry offers an equally valuable path that aligns with these same aspirations. Dentistry is a profession that blends science, artistry, and hands-on work, providing a powerful way to improve patients' lives by enhancing their health, confidence, and comfort. It's said that "Success is not the key to happiness. Happiness is the key to success." With this mindset, dentistry can become an exciting, fulfilling journey all on its own.

Consider the unique role dentists play. Far beyond just "fixing teeth," dentistry gives you the opportunity to impact patients' overall well-being. Oral health affects every part of a person's life—from their ability to eat comfortably to their self-confidence in social settings. Dentists often help people overcome deep-rooted fears and, in doing so, transform their attitudes toward healthcare. A friend of mine once told me, "Dentistry is where I see fear and relief coexisting." As a dentist, you'll have the chance to help people let go of that fear and feel better about their health. This work brings its own sense of reward and purpose—one that's deeply personal and essential.

I remember the first time I held a dental handpiece; it felt almost like holding a fine-tipped brush. The precision needed to perform a simple restoration made me realize that dentistry is as much an art as it is a science. One of my senior classmates described his first successful restoration as a "Eureka moment," a blend of skill and artistry he hadn't considered initially. He told me, "It was the first time I felt like a true healthcare provider, someone who could directly and immediately impact another person's life." This realization is what often transforms the perception of dentistry from a "fallback" option to a highly respected, deeply satisfying career.

Dentistry also offers endless opportunities for growth and exploration. There are numerous specializations within the field—pediatric dentistry, orthodontics, endodontics, and more. Each area combines medicine, skill, and artistry in unique ways, often igniting a passion many students didn't even realize they had. Shadowing a dentist or reading stories from practicing professionals can provide insight into what makes this profession special. Learning about their journeys may spark your own excitement, helping shift your perspective from "what could have been" to "what can be."

In many ways, dentistry requires a unique blend of strengths. It challenges you to be precise, creative, and compassionate. It allows you to master fine motor skills, think on your feet, and, ultimately, offer life-changing care to your patients. As you learn to master new techniques, you'll see that dentistry isn't a "second choice"—it's a path of its own, rich with potential and impact. Think of it as a shift in purpose, not a plan B, because as the proverb goes, "Every cloud has a silver lining." Dentistry may lead you toward a sense of fulfilment and accomplishment that rivals any achievement in medicine.

So, embrace dentistry not as a fallback but as an exploration of your talents in a field that needs skilled, compassionate practitioners. It is a career that not only holds purpose but allows you to continuously learn, adapt, and evolve.

Set New Goals within Dentistry

Setting new goals can reinvigorate your enthusiasm and provide a sense of direction within this new field. Dentistry is a vast profession with numerous specialties, each offering its own challenges and rewards. Take time to explore the areas that truly excite you, whether it's the precision and creativity of restorative procedures, the artistry of aesthetic dentistry, or the complexity and hands-on nature of oral surgery. By honing in on a specific interest, you'll find a renewed sense of purpose that makes every lecture, lab, and late-night study session feel worthwhile.

For instance, let's say you're drawn to restorative dentistry. This area allows you to help patients regain functionality and confidence, especially for those who may have struggled with damaged or missing teeth. Your goal could be to learn the most advanced techniques in dental restoration, ultimately allowing you to provide treatments that are durable, comfortable, and aesthetically pleasing. Perhaps you aim to master procedures like crowns, bridges, and implants, or become skilled at using CAD/CAM technology to design precise, customized solutions for patients.

Or maybe you're captivated by the potential of aesthetic dentistry, which is all about helping patients achieve smiles they're proud of. This path involves a deep understanding of both the science and artistry behind dental work. Setting goals in this field could involve learning advanced whitening techniques, veneers, and smile design principles. In helping people feel more confident about their smiles, you'll find both personal satisfaction and professional success.

If the adrenaline and precision of surgery excite you, oral surgery may be the direction to pursue. Here, your goals could include mastering the intricacies of surgical procedures, such as extractions, corrective jaw surgeries, or even reconstructive work. This field offers opportunities for ongoing learning, as surgical techniques and technologies are always evolving.

By setting specific goals within dentistry, you'll find yourself looking forward to classes, excited by the skills you're building, and proud of the progress you're making. Dentistry will become more than just a career—it'll be a passion that combines your interests, abilities, and dedication into something truly impactful. So, take time to explore, find your niche, and allow your goals to guide you forward.

Focus on the "Why" Behind Your Goals

If your dream was to make a difference in people's lives, dentistry offers a powerful way to fulfill that purpose. Many people see dentistry as "fixing teeth," but it's so much more than that. It's about restoring health, confidence, and well-being. I remember an instructor sharing a story about one of her first patients—a man who'd stopped smiling years ago because he was embarrassed by the state of his teeth. She worked with him to restore his smile, and months later, he sent her a heartfelt letter saying she'd given him back his life. That simple but profound impact solidified her sense of purpose in the field and made her realize just how deeply dentistry touches lives. In moments like these, it becomes clear that the true value of dentistry lies in the joy and confidence it restores to others.

Focus on the Skills You'll Gain and the Lives You'll Impact

Sometimes, the best way to overcome disappointment is to focus on what you can achieve moving forward. Dental school will teach you skills that are both empowering and impactful. You'll develop precision and patience as you work with tools that require meticulous attention to detail. You'll gain a deep understanding of the connection between oral health and overall wellness, which will allow you to educate and advocate for your patients' broader health. Imagine the satisfaction of helping a patient who has been in pain for months or the joy of restoring someone's confidence after years of hiding their smile. Each interaction reinforces the invaluable role you play in people's lives, turning initial setbacks into motivation.

Focus on What Makes You Unique

Your journey into dentistry, including the challenges you've faced, is what makes you unique. Not everyone takes a straight path to their goals; some of the most fulfilling journeys take a few unexpected turns. Coming into the field with your specific background adds versatility and resilience to your perspective. The experience of striving, falling short, and picking yourself back up will give you qualities like grit, empathy, and adaptability—all traits that will not only make you a better student but also a more understanding and compassionate practitioner.

In dental school, you'll find that your resilience becomes a strength. One of my classmates, who had initially struggled with not getting into medical school, shared how that experience helped him connect better with his patients. He would always take an extra moment to reassure patients, knowing firsthand what it felt like to overcome doubt. The proverb "Smooth seas do not make skillful sailors" perfectly sums up this mindset. It's these challenges that prepare you for the rewarding work you'll do in the future.

In dentistry, you have the chance to shape your own path, impact lives in a tangible way, and gain invaluable skills that go far beyond technical knowledge. By focusing on the "why" behind your goals and embracing what makes your journey unique, you'll find that dentistry isn't just a profession; it's an opportunity to make a lasting difference.

Setting New Goals and Embracing the Journey Ahead

One of the most empowering ways to overcome disappointment is to set small, achievable goals in this new chapter. Focusing on milestones—whether it's mastering a technique, acing an exam, or simply building camaraderie with classmates—will make each day feel purposeful. Each success, no matter how small, adds a layer of confidence and reminds you that this path is filled with its own unique rewards.

I'll never forget my first cavity filling on a practice mannequin. My hands were trembling as I went through the motions, and I couldn't believe how much time I'd spent studying technique only to feel like a beginner all over again. But when I finished, the sense of accomplishment was undeniable—it wasn't perfect, but it was a start. That small victory gave me a whole new respect for the precision and care dentistry demands, and it sparked a sense of pride that made me excited to learn more.

It's often in these early successes that our motivation begins to grow. One of my peers, who shared the same doubts after not getting into medical school, had a similar experience during a community outreach program. At first, she was unsure about the field, but seeing the grateful smiles of patients receiving care changed her perspective. That outreach experience, one she might never have had in medical school, became her turning point. She realized just how impactful hands-on work could be, and it helped her let go of past disappointments to fully embrace her role in dentistry.

Celebrate Small Wins and Find New Passions

Every step forward, no matter how small, is worth celebrating. Setting and achieving goals along the way is essential not only to building confidence but to discovering aspects of dentistry that you may not have initially considered. There's a Chinese proverb that says, "A journey of a thousand miles begins with a single step." That's the essence of dental school: each skill mastered and each patient helped becomes another step in your journey toward a meaningful career.

So embrace this chapter and set your sights on what you can accomplish right now. By celebrating each small win, you'll begin to see the beauty in the path you've chosen. In time, these early accomplishments will string together into a tapestry of growth, fulfillment, and purpose that feels wholly your own. Embracing this journey wholeheartedly turns what may have once felt like a detour into a destination full of new passions and possibilities.

Build Connections with Those Who Understand the Journey

You're not the first, nor will you be the last, to face a redirection in your academic path, and that shared experience can be a powerful source of comfort. Many dental students have found themselves initially disappointed, even disheartened, when life took them on a different path than they planned. But by reaching out to peers, mentors, and instructors who have also taken these unexpected turns, you'll find encouragement, perspective, and camaraderie that make moving forward a little easier. In fact, you may soon realize that many dental professionals who faced setbacks ended up finding pride and fulfillment in their work, transforming a perceived detour into a destination all its own.

One classmate, Nisha, went through this experience firsthand. She used to dread family gatherings, knowing that at some point, a relative would ask, "So, why didn't you go into medicine?" At first, these questions stung, serving as constant reminders of what she hadn't achieved. But as she opened up to her classmates about her journey, she discovered that she wasn't alone. Many of us had gone through similar experiences of having to adjust our expectations and forge new goals. Eventually, we created a small support group, meeting every week to share stories, frustrations, and successes. Those sessions became a source of strength—places where we could laugh, vent, and lean on each other. There's an old African proverb that says, "If you want to go fast, go alone; if you want to go far, go together." Building this network made each of us stronger, and our connections became a lifeline through the challenges of dental school.

Surround Yourself with a Supportive Network

Having people around you who believe in you can make a world of difference. Whether it's classmates who understand the daily demands of dental school, family members cheering on your efforts, or mentors offering guidance and wisdom, a supportive network helps you stay grounded. Sharing your journey with those who are going through similar challenges can build a sense of camaraderie. There's comfort in knowing that you're not alone on this path; others have faced these same struggles, and many have come out stronger and more passionate than ever.

Creating a network of supportive friends, mentors, and fellow students reminds you that your journey is valid, and there's no "wrong" way to reach your goals. Even the most winding roads can lead to meaningful destinations, and together, you can turn those shared moments of frustration, doubt, and triumph into a journey you're proud of. By connecting with others who've walked similar paths, you build a solid foundation to help you through the challenges and successes that lie ahead, reminding you every step of the way that this journey is yours to embrace.

A New Perspective on Success

The journey you're on is uniquely yours, and missing out on one goal doesn't equate to failure. Sometimes, it's the unexpected paths that shape our lives in ways we'd never imagined. I remember speaking with a seasoned dentist who shared that he'd originally aimed for medical school, and the detour into dentistry felt like a consolation prize at first. Yet, years later, he couldn't imagine his life any other way. Dentistry allowed him to impact people's lives in ways that felt personal, lasting, and fulfilling. "I didn't end up where I planned," he said, "but I ended up exactly where I belong."

This sentiment is echoed by countless dentists who began with dreams that led elsewhere. Dentistry may not have been your original vision, but it offers a chance to create a career that's both impactful and deeply rewarding. With every patient interaction, each skill you master, and each small victory, you'll see that you're building a career worth celebrating. The sting of missed opportunities will fade, and in time, you might find yourself grateful for the path that led you here. As the saying goes, "Success is not the key to happiness. Happiness is the key to success." If you find joy and fulfillment in your work, success will naturally follow.

Transforming Your Journey into Motivation

This new path is more than a detour—it's an opportunity to redefine success on your own terms. Every patient you help, every new technique you learn, and each challenge you face will enrich your journey and, in turn, the lives of those you touch.

Dentistry is a field that blends technical skill with compassion, allowing you to make tangible improvements in others' lives.

One peer of mine shared a similar story. She had initially been disappointed to end up in dental school rather than medical school, but during a volunteer clinic, she worked with a patient who had been in chronic pain due to untreated dental issues. After providing relief, the patient's gratitude was overwhelming. That experience changed her perspective. She realized that, as a dentist, she could transform lives in ways she had never anticipated.

Sometimes, it's the paths we don't initially choose that teach us the most about ourselves. They reveal strengths and passions we might never have discovered otherwise. By embracing this chapter, you'll open doors to accomplishments, relationships, and discoveries that make the journey truly worthwhile. There's a Japanese proverb that says, "Fall seven times, stand up eight." This speaks to the resilience and adaptability you're cultivating, qualities that will serve you not just in school but throughout your career.

A Final Thought

Letting go of past disappointments is a process, and it takes time, patience, and a willingness to see your future with optimism. Embrace your journey with a sense of purpose, and allow yourself to feel proud of choosing dentistry. In the end, success isn't about the title you hold; it's about the difference you make in the lives of others. Dentistry provides every bit as much opportunity to make a profound impact as any other healthcare field—if you approach it with an open heart and a commitment to excellence.

Give yourself grace, celebrate each step forward, and take pride in the decision you've made. This path may be different from the one you initially envisioned, but with time, you may find it to be as fulfilling—if not more so—than you ever expected.

It's easy to dwell on what could have been, but focusing on your future in dentistry will help you shift from what didn't happen to what can still happen. Recognize the vast potential of your new path and the exciting opportunities ahead.

Chapter 1: Laying the Foundation

Starting dental school is like stepping onto a brand-new path—thrilling yet slightly intimidating. This chapter is about helping you begin strong by setting clear expectations, managing initial challenges, and building a solid foundation for success that will carry you through your program. It's easy to feel overwhelmed by the intensity of dental school right from the start. However, with the right mindset and strategies, you can transform those first tentative steps into a confident stride.

The First-Day Jitters

Picture this: it's your first day of dental school, and the room is buzzing with energy. Everyone around you seems confident—perhaps a little intimidating. I vividly remember my first day, sitting in the lecture hall, heart racing as our professor introduced the rigorous curriculum. I fumbled with my notebook, feeling like a fish out of water. But then, the professor shared a piece of wisdom that put us all at ease: "You're not here because you're perfect. You're here to become skilled and resilient, and that's a process." Those words felt like a weight lifted off my shoulders. In that moment, I realized I wasn't alone in my uncertainty; we were all on this journey together.

Start Small, Dream Big

As the Chinese proverb goes, "A journey of a thousand miles begins with a single step." In dental school, that first step often involves managing expectations. Many students enter with high hopes but quickly discover that the workload is intense and success requires more than just intelligence; it demands resilience, time management, and self-discipline. The key is to pace yourself. Focus on one class, one project, or one skill at a time. Starting small, with manageable goals, allows you to grow steadily, gaining confidence with each accomplishment. Remember, the student who takes steady steps often goes further than one who tries to sprint through the journey.

Embracing the Surprises

One of the most surprising aspects of those early weeks is realizing that dental school isn't solely about teeth. You're delving into overall health, understanding how oral health connects to the rest of the body, and developing the dexterity to perform precise work under pressure. I felt this realization hit me during one of our first labs, where we practiced drilling on a mannequin. Nervous, I picked up the dental drill, my hands shaking with apprehension. I worried I wouldn't be able to keep my hand steady enough to perform the task. Yet, with each small success—whether it was drilling a cavity or placing an impression mold—I began to build a foundation of confidence.

Managing Expectations and Building Habits

Success in dental school comes from having realistic expectations. It's a marathon, not a sprint. Think of it as constructing a house: the foundation must be strong, and each brick laid carefully, even if it takes time. Develop habits that keep you focused—whether it's setting a schedule, carving out dedicated study time, or establishing a routine that includes moments for rest. You'll learn that getting through dental school isn't about constant hard work; it's about consistency, balance, and   persistence.

Transitioning to Dental School

Transitioning to dental school can feel overwhelming initially. The curriculum is vast, covering everything from basic sciences to intricate clinical techniques, and it's easy to feel lost in the details. The key is to understand the structure of your studies; this is crucial for managing both your time and mental health. When I started, I felt like I was swimming in a sea of information, but then I discovered the value of creating a roadmap for my courses and exams. A visual layout of what to expect helped reduce my anxiety and improved my focus. As the saying goes, "A goal without a plan is just a wish." By mapping out my journey, I turned those wishes into achievable milestones.

Understanding the Curriculum

The breadth of the curriculum can be both exciting and daunting. You'll dive into subjects like anatomy, pharmacology, and pathology, but you'll also spend countless hours honing your practical skills in the lab. That initial fear transforms into a determination to master each skill, proving to yourself that you are capable of more than you had believed.

Getting into the Mindset of a Dental Student

To truly succeed, you must cultivate the mindset of a dental student—a blend of discipline, resilience, and curiosity. There will be long nights spent poring over textbooks, studying anatomical diagrams, or practicing techniques until your hands ache. I recall battling against time, fuelled by caffeine and the unwavering belief that each hour spent studying would pay off. Yet, amid the challenges, moments of joy and fulfillment make it all worthwhile.

When clinic days rolled around, the excitement was palpable. The first time I worked with an actual patient, the nervous energy was electric. I remember standing at the entrance, heart pounding, knowing this was my chance to apply everything I had learned. As I greeted my patient, I felt a surge of purpose. That blend of nerves and exhilaration became a reminder of why I chose this path in the first place.

Building Resilience

Building resilience is crucial in dental school. You will encounter frustrations—difficult lab assignments, challenging exams, and moments when you feel like giving up. I faced my share of setbacks, especially during my initial attempts at performing complex procedures. I learned the hard way that mistakes are part of the process, and it's essential to embrace them rather than shy away. As the proverb says, "Fall seven times, stand up eight." Each stumble became a stepping stone, teaching me valuable lessons about patience and perseverance.

In those challenging moments, I found comfort and camaraderie among my classmates. We bonded over shared frustrations, late-night study sessions, and the triumphs we celebrated together, no matter how small. This sense of community became an anchor, reminding me that I wasn't alone on this journey.

Final Thoughts

As you embark on your dental school journey, remember that every day is an opportunity to learn and grow. Transitioning to this new phase will challenge you, but it will also shape you into a skilled professional who can make a difference in the lives of others. Embrace the process, acknowledge your fears, and celebrate your victories—both big and small. This chapter is just the beginning of a remarkable journey, and with each step, you're building not just a career, but a lifetime of purpose and fulfillment.

The first chapter of dental school is about finding your footing, learning the ropes, and realizing that every struggle is part of the process. As the African saying goes, "Smooth seas do not make skillful sailors." The challenges you face in these early months will teach you lessons that extend far beyond textbooks. They'll build the resilience, patience, and determination you'll need for the journey ahead. With each new day, as you overcome nerves, balance new knowledge, and celebrate small victories, you're laying a solid foundation—one that will help you become not only a competent dentist but a compassionate one too.

So, welcome to dental school. The journey may be long, but remember, the road is walked one step at a time. Embrace each day, learn from every challenge, and know that with each new skill, you're building a foundation for a rewarding career—and a lifetime of meaningful work.

Chapter 2: The Foundations of Effective Study

Starting Strong: Setting Up for Success

Embarking on your dental school journey is akin to laying the groundwork for a grand edifice; the strength and durability of what follows depend on how solidly you build that foundation. As you step into this vibrant yet challenging new world, it's essential to establish effective study routines tailored to the dense material you'll encounter. This can be both exciting and daunting, and the path to success requires careful planning and a proactive mindset.

Building that solid foundation for success right from the start involves more than just showing up to class and reading textbooks. It requires a strategic approach that balances theory and practice from day one. The intricacies of dentistry demand that you not only understand complex concepts but also develop practical skills that will serve you in the clinic. This means dedicating time to hands-on practice while ensuring you grasp the theoretical underpinnings of your work.

One of the keys to navigating this journey successfully is setting achievable goals. By breaking down your ambitions into manageable tasks, you'll find it easier to track your progress and celebrate small victories along the way. Whether it's mastering a new dental procedure or acing a particularly challenging exam, these milestones will build your confidence and reinforce your commitment to your studies.

Remember, as the old saying goes, "A journey of a thousand miles begins with a single step." Each step you take in these early years shapes the skilled professional you will become. By prioritizing effective study habits and focusing on both your theoretical knowledge and practical skills, you'll be better equipped to tackle the challenges ahead, laying the groundwork for a successful and fulfilling career in dentistry. Embrace this journey with an open heart and a curious mind, and you'll find that the effort you put into building your foundation will pay dividends throughout your time in dental school and beyond.

The First Steps in Study Routines

Embarking on your dental school journey can often feel overwhelming, like trying to sail through a vast ocean of knowledge without a compass. I vividly remember my early days in dental school, when the sheer volume of information felt daunting, with lectures, textbooks, and practical sessions all clamouring for my attention. One particularly enlightening moment came when a senior student shared a piece of wisdom that resonated deeply: "If you can't explain it simply, you don't understand it well enough." This insight became a turning point for me, illuminating the path to effective study routines. I learned that simplifying complex concepts not only made them easier to grasp but also built my confidence.

Creating a Comprehensive Study Schedule

One of the first steps to establishing an effective study routine is to create a comprehensive study schedule. Here's how to do it effectively:

Gathering Your Resources

As you embark on your journey through dental school, one of the first and most crucial steps is to gather all your resources. This process sets the foundation for effective study habits and time management, enabling you to visualize your responsibilities and commitments clearly. Let's delve into how you can organize your resources, along with practical examples that will resonate with your experiences as a dental student.

1. Your Roadmap to Success – Collecting and Using Course Syllabi

Starting a new term in dental school can be both exciting and overwhelming, with new courses, assignments, and responsibilities. To get a strong start, the first thing I recommend is gathering all the syllabi for your courses. These documents are your semester roadmap, detailing everything from course objectives and grading criteria to assignment deadlines and exam dates. In my own experience as a dental student, I found that organizing these syllabi at the outset not only provided clarity but also empowered me to manage my workload effectively, turning an intimidating semester into something more manageable.

At the beginning of each term, I would print out the syllabi for every class. Having a physical copy meant I could annotate, highlight, and quickly refer back to it whenever I needed. This practice wasn't just for convenience—it was about getting a tangible sense of my workload. By laying the syllabi out on my desk, I could immediately see what each course would demand.

One semester, I was taking Anatomy, Physiology, and Pharmacology simultaneously, all of which required intense memorization and understanding. I remember laying out each syllabus and realizing that two major exams, one in Anatomy and another in Pharmacology, were scheduled just days apart. The syllabi became my early warning system, helping me avoid the all-too-common pitfall of cramming last minute. I could see at a glance that I needed to begin reviewing earlier for those two classes. Knowing what was coming up gave me a head start, allowing me to create a study schedule that worked rather than one that stressed me out.

2. Highlight Key Dates and Requirements

Once I had my syllabi in hand, the next step was to go through each one, highlighting important dates, topics, and assessment types. This was more than just a formality; it was the first layer of active engagement with the course material. By highlighting these key details, I could see not only when assignments were due but also how they connected to each topic. This step helped me visualize the big picture and understand the progression of each course.

In Dental Materials, a course with hands-on practical sessions, I highlighted each lab session and associated readings. I knew that if I came to class unprepared, I would struggle to keep up with the hands-on work. One semester, we had a practical assessment on restorative materials the week after an exam in Dental Anatomy. By highlighting and noting these dates, I could plan study blocks specifically for the lab sessions and practical assessments, without sacrificing time for my theory exams. This proactive approach meant I didn't miss any deadlines and had ample time for each requirement.

3. Use Your Syllabi as a Planning Tool

Think of your syllabi as more than static documents—they're dynamic tools you can use to shape your study schedule. After reviewing and highlighting each syllabus, I would input the major deadlines, exams, and assignments into a calendar, creating a high-level view of my term. This big-picture approach helped me structure my weekly and daily study schedules to align with the demands of each course.

One challenging term involved extensive lab work and frequent quizzes in Oral Pathology, alongside heavy theoretical courses like Physiology. By mapping out all due dates on a single calendar, I could allocate more time for reading-intensive courses earlier in the semester and shift my focus to lab work as those deadlines approached. This allowed me to stay flexible, prioritizing each subject at the right time, rather than being blindsided by a last-minute assignment or quiz. Knowing what was coming up gave me a sense of control, which was crucial in such a high-pressure environment.

4. Recognize High-Impact Weeks and Plan Ahead

In dental school, certain weeks inevitably carry a heavier load—perhaps two midterms in the same week or a lab practical immediately following an exam. By pinpointing these "high-impact weeks" early on, I could prepare in advance, avoiding the stress that comes from scrambling at the last minute.

During my second semester, I had a particularly intense period with back-to-back exams in Physiology and Microbiology. By reviewing my syllabi, I noticed that the week before these exams was relatively light in terms of other responsibilities. So, I used that time to start preparing intensively for both exams, spreading out my study sessions to avoid burnout. Thanks to this advance planning, I was able to cover all necessary material and enter exam week feeling prepared rather than overwhelmed.

5. Use Color-Coding to Keep Everything Organized

Color-coding has become a popular organizational method for a reason—it works! Assigning each subject a color, both on my calendar and in my planner, allowed me to differentiate at a glance. For example, I used blue for Anatomy, green for Physiology, and yellow for labs. This color-coding gave me a visual layout that made it easy to spot patterns or clusters of assignments.

My color-coded calendar became an indispensable tool. On days when I had a full lab schedule, I'd see blocks of yellow filling up my calendar. This visual cue reminded me that I needed to set aside time in the preceding days to review lab notes and practice techniques. For major exams in Pharmacology (coded in purple), I would reserve specific purple blocks on the calendar, dedicating uninterrupted study sessions for that subject alone. This way, I never missed an important date or overlooked any requirement, and the colors made my calendar easy and enjoyable to use.

6. Regularly Update and Adjust as Needed

As the semester unfolds, new assignments, projects, and exams will inevitably pop up. To stay on top of everything, I made it a habit to review my syllabi and calendar every Sunday evening. This weekly check-in helped me ensure I was on track, adjust my study plan if necessary, and mentally prepare for the week ahead.

One week, I noticed that my calendar was unusually packed with quizzes and assignments. After reviewing my syllabi, I realized I'd need to adjust my schedule to fit in additional review time. This foresight prevented unnecessary stress and kept me in control of my workload. Having this "recalibration" each week kept me grounded, allowing me to focus on what mattered most in the moment without losing sight of the bigger picture.

Collecting and organizing your syllabi may seem like a small step, but it's an essential one. By treating your syllabi as living documents, engaging with them regularly, and using them as a foundation for your study schedule, you'll set yourself up for a productive and manageable semester. With every deadline mapped out and every lab session anticipated, you can confidently tackle the challenges of dental school, one step at a time.

Building Your Foundation with a Centralized Calendar

As a dental student, managing a packed schedule of lectures, labs, exams, and extracurriculars can feel overwhelming. That's where a centralized calendar comes in—it's more than just a tool; it's your roadmap for navigating the semester with confidence and control. By gathering everything you need into one accessible place, you can stay on top of your responsibilities, reduce stress, and free up mental space for learning and growth.

1. Choosing the Right Calendar Format

The first step in creating a centralized calendar is deciding whether to go digital or stick with a physical planner. Each has its advantages: a physical planner offers the satisfaction of crossing off completed tasks, while a digital calendar is flexible, with features like reminders and syncing across devices.

I used Google Calendar because it syncs across my phone and laptop, meaning I could always check my schedule, even between classes or on my way to the clinic. Setting reminders for exams and lab reports meant I was less likely to forget upcoming tasks, even during the busiest weeks. This saved me from the last-minute panic that often hits when you realize you've forgotten an assignment due the next morning.

2. Color-Coding for Organization and Clarity

Color-coding your calendar is a powerful tool for staying organized. Assigning each course and activity a different colour not only makes your calendar visually appealing but also allows you to assess your week at a glance.

I used blue for Anatomy, green for Physiology, and orange for extracurriculars. One semester, I had a challenging week with back-to-back exams in Anatomy and Physiology, plus a clinical workshop. Having these events color-coded helped me immediately spot which subjects I needed to prioritize. I could see that my week was dominated by Anatomy and Physiology, so I scheduled extra study blocks and reviewed notes for those courses in advance. When a friend invited me to a study session, I could easily decide whether I had time or needed to prioritize other commitments.

3. Inputting Key Dates and Deadlines

After setting up your calendar, start by entering all the key dates from each syllabus: exams, assignment deadlines, practicals, and presentations. This gives you an overview of critical periods, so you can allocate study time in advance rather than being blindsided.

Early in my first term, I noticed that my Anatomy and Biochemistry exams were scheduled just two days apart. Knowing this in advance allowed me to divide my study time carefully. I started with Dental materials well ahead of the exam date, and then focused on Anatomy closer to the test. By mapping out my study blocks, I avoided cramming and reduced stress, knowing I was prepared for both exams.

4. Adding Lab Sessions and Clinical Commitments

In dental school, labs and clinics require time and preparation, especially when dealing with complex procedures and equipment. Adding each lab session or clinical rotation to your calendar, along with reminders, can help you arrive prepared and makes the most of these hands-on experiences.

I had weekly labs in Restorative Dentistry to practice tooth-preparation techniques. Every Wednesday evening, I scheduled a reminder to review my notes and prepare any materials I'd need. This pre-lab routine meant I arrived prepared and ready to practice new techniques, rather than scrambling to understand procedures on the spot. Over time, I found that I was able to focus more on improving my skills than on catching up with the material.

5. Blocking Study Time and Including Self-Care

Creating dedicated blocks for studying each subject is essential to stay on top of your workload. By designating these blocks in advance, you're setting aside focused time that helps you prevent procrastination. But it's also important to schedule self-care—whether that's a coffee break, a workout, or a quiet evening to recharge. Taking time to rest can improve focus and help you avoid burnout.

I dedicated two hours every Tuesday evening to Anatomy, knowing that I found the subject challenging and needed extra time. I also reserved Friday afternoons for Pharmacology review. Self-care time was equally important, so I blocked out Saturday mornings to relax, grab a coffee, or go for a short run. Having self-care "appointments" reminded me that rest was part of my success strategy, helping me feel recharged and ready to tackle the next week.

6. Setting Reminders and Notifications

Setting reminders for assignments, exams, and labs is crucial to stay on track. Notifications serve as gentle nudges, prompting you to start projects early or check in on your progress well before a deadline.

For a major Oral Pathology project, I set reminders a week, three days, and one day before the due date. The first reminder prompted me to begin researching, the second to start drafting, and the last to finalize edits. By breaking the project into steps with layered reminders, I could stay on schedule without scrambling at the last minute. By the time the final reminder went off, I was calmly reviewing my finished work instead of rushing to complete it.

7. Weekly Reviews and Adjustments

A centralized calendar is a living document; it needs weekly attention to adapt to new commitments and challenges. Set aside a specific time each week to review and adjust your schedule. This allows you to catch any changes early and reallocate study blocks to meet new demands.

Every Sunday evening, I'd sit down with my calendar to review the upcoming week. This routine gave me a chance to shift study blocks or add time for assignments that were taking longer than expected. One week, I noticed that Dental Anatomy was proving to be more difficult than I had anticipated, so I added an extra study block on Thursday. This weekly check-in kept my schedule flexible, preventing any single class or project from throwing my entire week off balance.

A centralized calendar is more than just a scheduling tool—it's the foundation for navigating dental school with structure and confidence. By implementing simple strategies like color-coding, blocking study time, and setting reminders, you'll be able to prioritize your tasks and keep a healthy balance. Taking the time to regularly review and adjust your calendar ensures it remains a useful resource, one that supports you as you tackle the unique challenges of dental school. Whether you use a physical planner or a digital one, the goal is the same: a well-organized calendar can give you peace of mind and help you stay in control, so you can focus on excelling in your studies and building your clinical skills.

Organize Lab Schedules and Practicals

In dental school, lab sessions are pivotal for hands-on learning, so it's essential to keep track of your lab schedules. I remember dedicating a section in my planner specifically for lab-related activities. Each week, I would jot down what skills we would be practicing—whether it was crown preparations, root canal techniques, or extractions—and the materials I would need to prepare in advance.

For instance, if we had a lab session on tooth anatomy, I would ensure I had all my tools organized the night before. I even created a checklist of materials to bring: dental molds, instruments, and my lab journal. This way, I was never caught off guard and could focus on learning rather than scrambling to find my supplies.

Incorporate Extracurricular Commitments

As you gather your resources, don't forget to include any extracurricular commitments you may have. Participating in student organizations, volunteering for community outreach programs, or attending workshops can greatly enhance your educational experience. However, these activities also require time and energy, so it's crucial to factor them into your schedule.

During my time in dental school, I was involved in a few clubs, including the Dental Student Association and a community service initiative. I made it a point to add these events to my calendar as well, often setting reminders for meetings or project deadlines. By doing so, I was able to balance my academic responsibilities with extracurricular involvement, ensuring I didn't overcommit myself.

Utilize Digital Tools for Efficiency

In today's digital age, leveraging technology can streamline your resource gathering and organization. I found several apps that helped me manage my time and tasks effectively. For instance, apps like Todoist or Trello allowed me to create to-do lists and project boards. I could break down larger tasks, such as preparing for an exam, into manageable steps, tracking my progress along the way.Additionally, using cloud storage services like Google Drive or Dropbox allowed me to store and organize important documents and notes digitally. I created folders for each course, keeping all related materials in one accessible location. This way, I could easily find lecture notes, assignments, and supplementary resources whenever I needed them.

Review and Adjust Regularly

Finally, it's important to regularly review and adjust your gathered resources. As you progress through the semester, new assignments and commitments will arise. I made it a habit to set aside time at the beginning of each week to review my calendar and to-do lists. This practice helped me stay on top of my workload and adjust my study plans as needed.

For example, if I noticed that an exam was approaching and my study schedule was packed, I would shift my focus to prioritize revision for that subject. This proactive approach not only kept me organized but also reduced the stress that often accompanies the unpredictable nature of dental school.

Gathering your resources is a foundational step in achieving academic success in dental school. By collecting syllabi, creating a centralized calendar, organizing lab schedules, incorporating extracurricular activities, utilizing digital tools, and reviewing regularly, you can effectively visualize your responsibilities and manage your time. Remember, the key is not just to collect information but to make it work for you—turning potential chaos into a well-structured plan that supports your journey toward becoming a skilled dental professional. Embrace this process, and you'll find yourself more prepared and confident as you navigate the challenges ahead!

The Power of Setting Specific Study Blocks for Dental Students

In dental school, where dense information and complex concepts are the norm, effective studying isn't about cramming—it's about studying smartly. One technique that can be incredibly helpful in maintaining focus and improving retention is setting specific study blocks. By structuring your study time into short, focused bursts, you can avoid burnout, boost productivity, and make the most of each session. Research supports the effectiveness of studying in focused blocks, showing that sessions of around 25-50 minutes, with short breaks in between, can enhance concentration and reduce mental fatigue.

1. The Pomodoro Technique: Why It Works

The Pomodoro Technique is one of the most popular methods for breaking up study time. It involves studying for 25 minutes, followed by a 5-minute break. After completing four 25-minute sessions (or "Pomodoros"), you take a longer break of around 15-30 minutes. This cycle of intense focus followed by brief breaks can improve mental stamina, helping you stay focused throughout even the longest study days.

When I first started using the Pomodoro Technique in my second year of dental school, I noticed a difference in my energy levels. Instead of feeling mentally drained after two hours of nonstop study, I felt refreshed and able to tackle more material. For example, I'd spend one 25-minute session reviewing nerve pathways for Neuroanatomy. After a quick 5-minute break (usually a stretch or a short walk), I'd move on to a different topic like tooth morphology for my next Pomodoro. This not only kept my mind fresh but also made each study session feel manageable, even on the busiest days.

2. Setting Specific Study Goals for Each Block

Simply sitting down for 25 minutes isn't enough—you need to know what you'll focus on during each block. Setting specific study goals keeps each session purposeful and gives you a clear sense of progress. These goals can be topic-specific (e.g., "master the mandibular nerve branches") or task-based (e.g., "summarize lecture notes on periodontal disease").

During a busy exam week, I divided my Pomodoros into precise objectives for each session. For instance, the first Pomodoro was dedicated solely to understanding the various stages of tooth development. I didn't let myself drift into other topics. In the next session, I'd focus entirely on practicing dental histology concepts. Keeping each block tightly focused prevented me from feeling overwhelmed by the sheer volume of material and helped me track my progress throughout the day.

3. Avoiding Burnout with Breaks

Dental school can be physically and mentally exhausting, and studying for long hours without breaks can lead to burnout. Regular short breaks give your brain a chance to recharge, reducing the risk of burnout and keeping you more engaged over time. Use breaks to get up, stretch, hydrate, or simply take a mental breather. You might feel guilty about "wasting time" on breaks, but they're essential for sustained productivity.

After a 25-minute session of memorizing pharmacology drug names, I'd take a 5-minute break to stand up, stretch, and get some fresh air. I found that when I returned to my notes, I could retain the information much better than if I had tried to power through without a break. My longer breaks, like the 15-30 minute one after four Pomodoros, became a chance to refresh completely, so I'd often go for a walk around campus, grab a snack, or do something that didn't require mental effort.

4. Adapting the Pomodoro Technique for Complex Topics

Some dental topics require deeper concentration, making it hard to cover them in just 25 minutes. For these, consider extending your study blocks to 50 minutes, with a 10-minute break afterward. This adjustment allows you to dive deeper into challenging material while still incorporating breaks to maintain your mental stamina.

When studying for my Dental Anatomy practical, I used 50-minute blocks instead of 25-minute ones because I needed more time to focus on understanding and sketching detailed tooth structures. I'd spend the entire session working on just one tooth and its unique anatomical features. Afterward, I'd take a longer, 10-minute break to refresh. This approach gave me the time needed to process the complexity of the material without feeling rushed, while still preventing mental exhaustion.

5. Using Your Breaks Wisely

How you spend your breaks matters. Avoid activities that might drain you mentally, like scrolling through social media or answering emails, as these can make it harder to refocus. Instead, engage in activities that allow your mind to rest and reset.

During my 5-minute breaks, I'd sometimes do breathing exercises, especially if I was feeling anxious about an upcoming test. Other times, I'd just stand by the window and let my mind wander or take a few minutes to drink water and move around. These simple activities made a huge difference, helping me feel more centered and ready for the next session.

6. Building Momentum with the Pomodoro Technique

One of the best things about the Pomodoro Technique is how it helps build momentum. Each time you complete a Pomodoro, you get a small sense of achievement, which can keep you motivated. Tracking completed Pomodoros, either in a journal or a digital tracker, allows you to look back and see how much you've accomplished, which can be a major confidence booster.

I kept a small journal to mark each completed Pomodoro. At the end of a long day, I'd see rows of completed study blocks and feel a real sense of achievement. This visual reminder of my hard work helped counter any doubts I had about my progress. If I completed 8 Pomodoros in a day, I knew I'd devoted nearly 4 solid hours to studying, plus essential break time. This helped me stay positive and motivated, even when the material felt challenging.

Structuring Your Study Time with Specific Blocks

In dental school, every bit of time counts, and learning to use it efficiently can be a game-changer. By setting specific study blocks, you're not just organizing your time—you're creating a system that supports both productivity and well-being. The Pomodoro Technique, with its structured balance of study and breaks, is a simple yet powerful way to tackle even the most demanding weeks. Whether you stick to 25-minute blocks or adapt to longer ones for certain subjects, remember that taking breaks is just as important as the study time itself. With practice, this technique will become a cornerstone of your study routine, allowing you to absorb material effectively and stay refreshed, focused, and prepared for the next step in your dental journey.

Maximizing Success in Dental School: The Importance of Regular Review Sessions and Flexibility in Your Study Schedule

In the demanding environment of dental school, it's easy to get caught up in constantly moving forward, tackling new material as it comes. However, true mastery requires more than just covering topics once and moving on. Regular review sessions and the willingness to adjust your study schedule as needed are essential practices for solidifying knowledge, managing your workload, and ultimately excelling in your courses.

1. The Power of Regular Review Sessions: Why Reinforcement Matters

When you're in dental school, each week brings a new influx of complex material—from intricate anatomical structures to complex biochemical processes. Without regular reinforcement, it's easy to forget what you learned a few days or weeks ago, which can lead to last-minute cramming and unnecessary stress during exam time. Incorporating review sessions into your schedule not only strengthens your understanding but also ensures that you retain the knowledge long-term.

I found that dedicating Sundays to review was a game-changer. I would go back over the material I had studied throughout the week, whether it was oral histology, anatomy, or physiology. Instead of passively reading, I actively engaged with the content—recreating diagrams from memory, summarizing key points, or testing myself with flashcards. This weekly review process prevented gaps in my knowledge from forming and meant I didn't have to relearn entire topics when exams approached. Over time, I noticed that I could recall details more effortlessly, which gave me a significant confidence boost, especially in high-pressure situations like clinical exams.

2. Creating a Review Plan that Works for You

Simply scheduling a review session isn't enough—having a structured approach for what to review and how to do it makes a big difference. Aim to cover a mix of recent material and older topics. This practice strengthens your understanding of foundational concepts and prepares you for cumulative exams, where knowledge from different modules often overlaps.

I found it helpful to divide my review sessions into focused segments. For instance, during one Sunday review, I would dedicate 30 minutes to summarizing the previous week's anatomy lectures and another 30 minutes to going over older pharmacology flashcards. Breaking the session down like this kept it engaging and ensured I wasn't neglecting any subject. By rotating through different topics in this way, I felt more confident that my understanding was well-rounded.

3. Adjusting Your Study Plan for Challenging Topics

In dental school, you'll inevitably encounter subjects that require more time and effort than others. Whether it's a challenging histology unit or a complex dental anatomy module, it's important to recognize when something needs extra attention and be flexible enough to adjust your schedule accordingly.

When I started studying histology, I quickly realized it was more challenging than I'd anticipated. The details of tissue structures and cellular arrangements took longer to grasp than I'd planned for. Rather than sticking rigidly to my original schedule, I decided to allocate extra time to histology on Monday and Thursday evenings, which helped me dive deeper into the subject without sacrificing my progress in other areas. I also found it helpful to reach out to classmates for study sessions or ask questions in our group chat. Making this adjustment early on prevented stress from building up and kept me on track with the rest of my coursework.

4. Building a Flexible Study Routine

Flexibility is one of the most underrated aspects of a successful study routine. A rigid schedule might seem like it will help you stay on track, but dental school requires adaptability. Your schedule should work for you—not the other way around. Building in room for adjustments ensures that you can address your needs in real time, whether that means devoting more time to a tough topic or taking an unexpected break to recharge.

During a particularly intense semester, I found myself struggling with unexpected projects and deadlines. Initially, I tried to stick to my original study plan, which ended up increasing my stress. Realizing that this wasn't sustainable, I adopted a more adaptable approach, where I prioritized my heaviest topics first and then adjusted my weekly goals based on how things went. If I covered my high-priority topics faster than expected, I used the extra time for lighter or supplemental material. On the other hand, if something took longer, I knew I had enough flexibility to shift around other tasks. This made my routine feel supportive rather than rigid, and I was able to keep my stress levels manageable.

5. Tracking Your Progress and Adjusting Regularly

Regularly assessing your progress and making adjustments to your schedule is critical. This can mean shifting your focus to different subjects as exams approach or adding more review time for topics you find particularly challenging. Think of your study plan as a living document that changes with your needs.

At the end of each week, I took a few minutes to reflect on how my study sessions went and where I was in terms of progress. For example, I might find that my pharmacology review sessions were going smoothly but that I was falling behind in pathology. Recognizing this early allowed me to allocate more time to pathology for the next week, ensuring that I didn't neglect any areas. I also kept a study journal where I'd jot down specific challenges I encountered, like memorizing drug interactions, which helped me adjust my approach proactively rather than waiting until I was under pressure before exams.

6. The Benefits of Embracing Flexibility and Regular Review

Together, regular review sessions and a flexible schedule create a balanced approach that supports both your short-term and long-term learning goals. By consistently reinforcing your knowledge and adjusting your plan as needed, you build a strong foundation that helps you stay on top of your studies without unnecessary stress. Embracing flexibility allows you to respond to challenges in real time, while regular review ensures that your understanding is thorough and lasting.

Dental school is a marathon, not a sprint. By incorporating weekly review sessions, you can reinforce what you've learned and prevent gaps in your knowledge, making exams and clinical assessments less daunting. A flexible schedule allows you to adapt to the demands of your coursework and personal needs, ensuring that your study plan is both effective and sustainable. These strategies not only help you succeed academically but also teach you how to manage a demanding workload with resilience and adaptability—a skill set that will serve you well in your dental career.

Mastering Complex Concepts in Dental School: A Guide to Simplifying Study Material

Dental school is filled with intricate and extensive material that can feel overwhelming at times. Whether you're diving into the layers of a tooth, understanding the nervous system, or memorizing pharmacology pathways, the depth and breadth of knowledge required demand a strategic approach. Once you've established a study schedule, the next crucial step is simplifying what you're learning. Breaking down complex concepts, using relatable analogies, teaching the material, and incorporating visual aids can help you transform complicated topics into clear and digestible knowledge. This approach not only helps you retain information better but also allows you to build a solid understanding that will support your journey as a dentist.

1. Breaking Down Topics: Making Information Manageable

When faced with a dense topic, tackling everything at once is daunting and can lead to confusion or shallow understanding. By breaking down a subject into smaller, manageable parts, you can focus on one element at a time, allowing for a more in-depth and steady accumulation of knowledge.

In dental anatomy, I initially felt overwhelmed by the sheer number of structures to learn. To make the information more approachable, I decided to focus on one section of the mouth at a time. I began with the maxilla and spent an entire day on the maxillary incisors alone. I drew detailed diagrams, labelled each part, and noted their specific characteristics and functions. This allowed me to fully digest the information before moving on to other areas, like the mandibular teeth. By tackling the content piece by piece, I built a foundation that was both solid and easy to expand upon as I moved forward. This approach made studying feel more manageable and boosted my confidence, knowing I was mastering each part thoroughly.

2. Using Analogies: Relating New Information to Familiar Concepts

Analogies can be a powerful tool to bridge the gap between unfamiliar concepts and what you already know. They make complex information feel more accessible, memorable, and often even intuitive by connecting it with everyday experiences.

When learning about the layers of a tooth, I found it difficult to remember each layer's properties and functions. To help, I began to think of the tooth like a layered cake: the enamel was the "outer frosting" that's hard and protective; the dentin was the "cake layer" underneath that provides structure; and the pulp, containing nerves and blood vessels, was the "filling" at the center. This analogy helped me remember both the structure and function of each layer, making the anatomy of a tooth easier to recall during exams.

Example for Physiology: Similarly, when studying the nervous system, I likened the network of nerves to a series of electrical cables, where the central nervous system acts as the main control hub. Signals travel along these "wires" to different parts of the body, and synapses serve as switches connecting various "cables." This analogy allowed me to visualize the transmission of information in a way that was easy to understand and recall. Making these connections helped transform abstract information into memorable images, enhancing my grasp of complex topics.

3. Teaching the Material: Deepening Your Understanding by Explaining to Others

Teaching a concept is one of the most effective ways to reinforce and solidify your knowledge. When you try to explain material in simple terms, it forces you to truly process and understand the information, highlighting any areas that need further clarification.

In my study group, I frequently volunteered to explain challenging topics, like the various types of oral mucosa. Preparing to teach required me to review and simplify the material, organizing it into digestible pieces. I created a mini-lecture and visual aids to present to my peers. By breaking down the characteristics of each mucosa type, I not only deepened my understanding but also gained insight from the questions and perspectives of my classmates. This technique became my go-to method for studying complex topics because it helped me reinforce my understanding and allowed me to help others in the process.

Even when studying alone, I would practice this method by explaining topics out loud as if I were teaching an audience. For instance, when studying the temporomandibular joint (TMJ), I pretended I was presenting to a class, detailing each part and its function. This "teaching to myself" approach revealed areas I hadn't fully grasped, giving me the chance to revisit and strengthen my understanding.

4. Using Visual Aids: Enhancing Retention Through Diagrams and Models

Visual aids are invaluable in dental school, especially for subjects like dental anatomy and physiology, where spatial understanding is critical. Diagrams, flowcharts, and 3D models can help turn abstract concepts into tangible representations, making them easier to grasp and remember.

When studying dental anatomy, I used clay to create small 3D models of various types of teeth. Each model represented a different structure, like incisors, canines, and molars, with their unique shapes and features. By handling these models, I developed a spatial understanding of tooth morphology, which later helped me in practical applications. This tactile approach made it much easier to visualize the teeth during exams and in the clinical setting.

I also relied heavily on diagrams and flowcharts for complex processes. For instance, I created a flowchart to illustrate blood circulation, tracing the path through the heart's chambers, into the lungs, and back to the body. When I was studying pharmacology, I drew out biochemical pathways step-by-step, adding colors and annotations. By visualizing these processes, I could better understand each step and its connection to the overall system, making intricate topics far easier to retain and recall.

Mastering complex information is key to a successful career in dentistry. By breaking down topics, using analogies, teaching others, and employing visual aids, you create a study process that is manageable, effective, and memorable. Simplifying concepts isn't just about easing the learning process—it's about developing a deep, intuitive understanding of the material that will serve you well throughout dental school and beyond. Implementing these strategies will help you tackle the challenges of dental school with confidence and clarity, setting you up for long-term success in your career.

Reflect and Review: The Power of Self-Assessment in Dental School

Reflecting and reviewing regularly is essential to mastering the intricate and demanding material in dental school. This practice not only reinforces what you've learned but also helps identify areas needing more attention. Consistent self-assessment builds your knowledge progressively, enhancing retention and comprehension over time. Here's how you can incorporate daily reflection, weekly reviews, and accountability into your routine.

1. Daily Reflection: Solidifying Today's Learning

Taking a few minutes each day to reflect on what you studied can significantly impact your learning process. This daily habit allows you to consolidate your knowledge, highlight key takeaways, and note any lingering questions that arose during your studies. By integrating reflection into your routine, you're better equipped to build a cumulative understanding of complex topics, especially in courses where new material builds on foundational knowledge.

When I first dove into oral pathology, the volume of information felt overwhelming. Each day, I set aside five minutes to review the main points I had covered, jotting down any lingering questions or concepts that didn't fully make sense. I maintained a small journal specifically for this purpose. For instance, after a lecture on differentiating between various types of cysts, I noted my struggles in distinguishing them. I marked it for clarification in my next study session. By regularly revisiting these points, I developed a stronger grasp of the material, minimizing the stress of cramming before exams.

Tip: Create a "Reflection Journal" for daily reviews. Dedicate a page each day to jot down three key elements: a crucial concept learned, a challenging topic, and a question that needs further exploration. This will not only keep track of your progress but also help you pinpoint areas that require additional focus.

2. Weekly Reviews: Building a Strong Foundation

Weekly reviews provide an opportunity to look at the broader picture, connecting various topics and reinforcing your memory. This practice is particularly beneficial in dental school, where each new lesson builds upon what you previously learned. Use this time to create condensed summaries of the week's material, as these summaries will serve as quick references and be especially useful for exam preparation.

Every Sunday, I allocated an hour to review my notes from the past week, creating summary sheets for each topic. For instance, during a week focused on pharmacology, I summarized key drugs, their mechanisms of action, and notable side effects.

Additionally, I included any relevant drug interactions or contraindications that might arise in clinical scenarios. This one-page summary became a crucial resource during exam prep, allowing me to quickly refresh my memory on essential principles without sifting through a mountain of notes. Establishing this weekly routine not only solidified my understanding but also boosted my confidence as I tackled new material.

Tip: Consider color-coding your summaries. For pharmacology, you might use different colours to highlight various drug classes, mechanisms, and side effects. This visual distinction will help categorize the information, making it easier to recall when needed.

3. Staying Accountable: Creating a Supportive Study Network

Having a study partner or mentor to hold you accountable can be a game-changer in your educational journey. Sharing your goals with someone else provides an extra layer of motivation and helps you stay on track. Regular check-ins not only maintain consistency in your study habits but also create a support system for navigating the challenges of dental school together.

I partnered with a classmate for weekly check-ins. Each Sunday, we'd discuss our study goals for the upcoming week. For example, I might set a goal to master the cranial nerves, while my partner focused on dental radiology. By sharing our objectives, we both felt more committed to achieving them. This mutual commitment fostered a sense of accountability, as I knew I had to report my progress to someone else. Our discussions also served as opportunities to share study tips, resources, and strategies. On particularly challenging weeks, we would encourage each other to stick to our goals, transforming study sessions from solitary tasks into collaborative, rewarding experiences.

> **Tip:** Schedule a weekly 15-minute call or meet up with a classmate or mentor to discuss your progress. Set two or three specific goals for the week and update each other on them during your check-in. This shared accountability structure can help keep you motivated and alleviate feelings of isolation during stressful times.

How to Implement a Reflect and Review Routine

By combining daily reflection, weekly reviews, and accountability, you can create a sustainable study routine that allows for gradual mastery of complex topics. Here's how to start:

Create a Routine: Allocate 5–10 minutes at the end of each day for reflection and an hour each week for review. Schedule these times consistently, treating them as important parts of your academic day.

Use Summaries: Develop a consistent format for your weekly summaries (e.g., bullet points, charts, or mind maps) so that you have a ready-to-use template each week. This will streamline the process and make it easier to capture essential information.

Find a Study Partner or Mentor: Reach out to a classmate or mentor, and suggest a weekly check-in. You don't have to study the same material; just sharing your goals can help maintain motivation and provide the support needed during difficult weeks.

The Long-Term Benefits of Reflection and Review

Incorporating a reflection and review routine into your study process can transform how you approach learning in dental school. Daily reflection builds consistency, weekly reviews reinforce memory, and accountability creates a supportive environment, keeping you engaged and motivated. By investing time in self-assessment, you're not just preparing for exams; you're laying the groundwork for a successful career in dentistry. This steady, reflective approach will help you retain what you learn and navigate complex material with greater ease and confidence.

By committing to this process, you'll find that your understanding deepens, making it easier to connect concepts and apply your knowledge in practical settings. This holistic approach to learning ensures you're not only academically prepared but also equipped with the skills necessary for a thriving dental practice.

As you progress through dental school, remember the wisdom in the proverb, "Failing to plan is planning to fail." A structured routine, along with proactive study techniques, transforms the overwhelming challenges of dental school into a manageable and rewarding journey. Each step you take lays the groundwork for your future as a skilled dental professional, shaping not just your knowledge base but also your confidence and competence.

With dedication and perseverance, you can navigate the ocean of knowledge ahead of you. Instead of feeling intimidated by the vast array of subjects, approach them as opportunities for growth and learning. Embrace the challenges, celebrate your achievements, and remain resilient in the face of obstacles. Your hard work today is an investment in your future career, and each small victory will propel you toward your ultimate goal: becoming a capable and compassionate dentist.

In summary, establishing effective study routines in dental school is about creating a plan, simplifying complex material, reflecting regularly, and maintaining a positive mindset. By embracing this structured approach, you will not only survive dental school but thrive in it, emerging as a knowledgeable and confident practitioner ready to make a difference in your patients' lives.

Concentrating During Lectures and Effective Note-Taking

Navigating the rigorous demands of dental school can sometimes feel like an uphill battle, particularly when faced with the deluge of information presented during lectures. However, mastering concentration and effective note-taking can significantly enhance your understanding and retention of material, setting you up for success. Below is a detailed guide filled with strategies and techniques drawn from personal experiences that helped me excel in my studies.

Cultivating Concentration in Lectures

1. Preparation is Key: Taking time to review relevant material before class can make a world of difference. This doesn't mean you need to memorize every detail; rather, familiarize yourself with key concepts. By skimming through lecture slides or required readings the night before, I was often able to identify areas I struggled with, allowing me to formulate questions and actively engage during class.

I vividly recall attending a lecture on oral pathology. After reviewing my notes the night before, I was able to connect various disease processes discussed in class with the concepts I had studied. This preparation transformed my experience from passive listening to an active pursuit of understanding.

2. Create a Comfortable Environment: Your physical surroundings can greatly influence your ability to concentrate. Choose a seat that minimizes distractions; for me, this meant sitting closer to the front where I could engage more easily with the lecturer. Arriving early to set up my laptop, notebooks, and any other materials helped establish a focused mindset. Sitting near the front also fostered a greater sense of accountability to participate actively.

3. Limit Distractions: In our digital age, distractions are everywhere, especially from smartphones. To combat this, I made it a habit to silence my phone and keep it out of sight during lectures. If I was using a laptop, I restricted myself from social media and unrelated websites. I learned the hard way that even a single glance at notifications could derail my focus for the rest of the session.

4. Practice Mindfulness: When your mind starts to wander, taking a moment to refocus can be incredibly beneficial. Techniques like deep breathing help ground you. For instance, before a lecture begins, I would take a few deep breaths to center my thoughts and set an intention for what I wanted to learn that day. This practice transformed my mindset, making me feel more present and engaged.

5. Active Listening: Approach lectures as an interactive experience. Nod, smile, and actively engage with the lecturer's points. Participating in discussions and asking questions keeps your mind sharp and prevents it from drifting. I found that treating lectures as conversations rather than monologues dramatically improved my retention.

6. Physical Engagement: Keep your body engaged to help your mind stay focused. Simple actions like taking notes, nodding in agreement, or doodling related diagrams can enhance concentration. When my professor discussed various types of teeth, I often sketched their shapes and functions, which not only kept me attentive but also deepened my understanding.

7. Short Breaks: If the lecture is lengthy, give yourself permission to take brief mental breaks. Stretching your legs or even just taking a deep breath can re-energize your mind. I would occasionally glance around the room to reorient myself, allowing my brain a moment to process the information before moving on.

Effective Note-Taking Techniques

1. Choose Your Method: Different note-taking methods cater to various learning styles. The Cornell Method, for instance, divides your page into three sections—cues, notes, and summary. I frequently utilized this method, especially during anatomy lectures, as it helped me highlight key terms and summarize the lecture content effectively.

Other methods include Outlining, where bullet points and indents organize information hierarchically, and Mapping, which uses diagrams to visually represent information. Mapping was particularly helpful in my studies, as it allowed me to see connections and processes clearly.

2. Be Selective: Rather than attempting to write down everything the lecturer says, focus on capturing key points, definitions, and examples. Develop a shorthand system of abbreviations or symbols that makes sense to you. For instance, I often used "DC" for dental caries, which allowed me to jot down notes swiftly without losing track of the lecture.

3. Highlight Key Concepts: Use colors to emphasize critical information. For example, I'd assign one color for definitions, another for examples, and a third for major points. This visual organization not only made my notes more appealing but also facilitated easier review later on. During a lecture on periodontal disease, I used a bright color to highlight treatment options, making that section easier to reference during study sessions.

4. Incorporate Visuals: Including diagrams, charts, and sketches can enhance your notes and make them more engaging. When learning about oral anatomy, I often drew simple diagrams alongside my notes to illustrate the positions of different teeth, reinforcing my understanding and making my notes visually appealing.

5. Ask Questions: If something isn't clear, jot down questions in your notes. This practice keeps you engaged and provides topics to explore further with peers or professors later. I found that writing down questions helped clarify my understanding and deepened my learning experience.

6. Review and Revise: After class, dedicate time to review your notes. Rephrasing complex points in your own words or adding insights from textbooks or discussions can enhance comprehension. I made it a routine to revisit my notes within 24 hours of the lecture to reinforce what I learned, filling in any gaps while the material was still fresh in my mind.

Preparing Your Own Notes from Textbooks

1. Skimming Before Reading: Prior to delving into a textbook chapter, skim it first. Examine headings, subheadings, and highlighted terms to get a sense of the structure and main ideas. This preliminary overview primes your brain for the details to come.

2. Chunking Information: Break the text into manageable sections. Instead of attempting to absorb an entire chapter at once, focus on one subsection at a time. I found that summarizing smaller chunks made retention easier and less overwhelming.

3. Summarization Techniques: As you read, take notes in your own words. This reinforces learning and fosters a deeper understanding of the material. After completing a section, write a brief summary at the end to consolidate your knowledge. For instance, after a challenging chapter on oral pathology, I would craft a summary focusing on the disease processes and their clinical implications.

4. Incorporate Visuals: Utilize diagrams, charts, and tables to represent complex information visually. For example, during anatomy studies, I often drew diagrams of structures, which helped me visualize their relationships and solidified my understanding.

5. Create a Study Guide: Compile your notes into a comprehensive study guide that includes essential definitions, concepts, and diagrams. This guide becomes an invaluable resource for exam preparation, helping you synthesize everything you've learned. Over time, I built a study guide that reflected the course content while incorporating my understanding of how different concepts interlinked.

6. Regularly Update Your Notes: As your studies progress, continually refine and enhance your notes. Incorporating new insights from lectures or practical experiences increases their value over time. I found that revisiting my notes weekly or bi-weekly helped me stay sharp on the material and identify areas needing further review.

Mastering concentration during lectures and employing effective note-taking techniques are crucial skills for success in dental school. By preparing ahead, actively engaging in class, and using strategic note-taking methods, you can transform your educational experience. Moreover, creating your own notes from textbooks not only aids retention but also fosters a deeper understanding of complex concepts.

Remember, learning is a journey, and every step you take to enhance your study habits brings you closer to becoming a proficient and confident dental professional. Embrace these techniques, adapt them to your style, and watch your academic performance soar!

Mastering Effective Study Techniques

Embarking on your dental school journey is akin to setting sail on an ocean filled with vast knowledge and numerous challenges. Traditional study methods often leave students adrift, struggling to grasp the depth of information required to excel in this rigorous field. Simply reading textbooks or passively listening to lectures may not yield the profound understanding you need. Instead, embracing active learning strategies can transform your study routine into a powerful ally for retention and comprehension. Let me share some effective study techniques that I found invaluable during my dental school experience, complete with practical examples to guide you in applying these methods to your studies.

Active Learning: Engage with Your Material

Active learning is about engaging deeply with the content rather than absorbing it passively. It involves immersing yourself in what you're learning through various means, such as discussing concepts with peers, teaching what you've learned, or applying theories to real-world scenarios. I vividly remember forming a study group during my first anatomy class. Every week, we met to quiz each other on the anatomy of the jaw, utilizing models and visual aids to reinforce our learning.

One memorable evening stands out: while we were reviewing the molars, someone hilariously misidentified a maxillary molar as a canine! The room erupted in laughter, and while it was a light-hearted moment, it reinforced a crucial lesson: camaraderie makes studying less daunting and infinitely more enjoyable. This shared experience not only enhanced our understanding of dental anatomy but also forged lasting friendships that supported us through the rigorous demands of dental school.

Another effective approach to active learning was role-playing during our oral pathology course. We simulated patient interactions, discussing symptoms and potential diagnoses, which solidified our understanding of complex conditions and prepared us for future patient encounters. These collaborative sessions were not only informative but also brought an element of excitement and unpredictability, reflecting real-life scenarios we would face in practice.

Memory Strategies: Visual and Rhythmic Techniques

Memorizing the intricate details of dental anatomy can sometimes feel like climbing a mountain without any gear—overwhelming and daunting. With the vast array of structures, functions, and terminologies to master, it's easy to feel lost. However, by utilizing effective memory strategies such as visual mnemonics and rhythmic techniques, you can transform this challenge into an engaging and enjoyable learning experience. I'd like to share some practical approaches that proved invaluable during my studies, accompanied by personal anecdotes that illustrate their effectiveness.

1. The Power of Visual Mnemonics: Bringing Information to Life

Visual mnemonics are potent tools that can help you retain complex information by associating it with vivid imagery. When faced with memorizing the cranial nerves, for instance, I decided to create a memorable character for each nerve. I imagined Olaf the Snowman for the Optic Nerve (II), envisioning him wearing oversized glasses to represent vision. This quirky image not only made the nerve easier to remember but also added a touch of humor to my study routine.

To further cement these associations, I took to drawing. I sketched simple cartoons or diagrams for each nerve. For example, I drew Olaf alongside a large eye, which helped create a visual anchor in my mind. Each time I needed to recall the cranial nerves, this mental picture of Olaf would pop into my head, triggering a cascade of information associated with that image. The effectiveness of this approach became clear during exams when I could easily recall not just the names but also the functions of the nerves.

2. Rhythmic Techniques: Making Memorization Fun

Music has a unique way of embedding information into our memories, and rhythmic techniques can make memorization much more enjoyable. I distinctly recall one evening when I was feeling overwhelmed with the cranial nerves. To lighten the mood, I decided to craft a catchy song set to a familiar tune. Using the melody of "Twinkle, Twinkle, Little Star," I created lyrics that outlined the names and functions of the cranial nerves:

"Olfactory, optic too,

Oculomotor, trochlear, woo!

Trigeminal, abducens,

Facial, vestibulocochlear, hence..."

This playful adaptation not only made studying enjoyable but also transformed a tedious memorization task into a fun sing-along. I found myself humming this tune in the days leading up to my exams, and the rhythm helped the information stick. Whenever I encountered an exam question on cranial nerves, I could hear the melody playing in my mind, guiding me to the right answers.

3. Hands-On Learning: Engaging Your Senses

Engaging multiple senses can significantly enhance memory retention. A technique I found particularly effective was hands-on practice. While studying tooth anatomy, I spent hours molding clay models of different teeth. This tactile experience was invaluable, as shaping and sculpting the clay helped me visualize the unique features of each tooth type—incisors, canines, premolars, and molars.

For instance, while creating a model of a maxillary first molar, I paid close attention to its distinct cusps and grooves, reminding myself of how these features contribute to mastication. As I worked, I recalled clinical relevance and function, solidifying my understanding through this engaging process. This multi-sensory approach—seeing, touching, and manipulating materials—created a deeper connection with the content that passive reading could never achieve.

4. Combining Visual Aids with Physical Models

Another strategy that greatly improved my spatial understanding was combining visual aids with physical models. When studying the maxillary sinus, I found it helpful to use both textbook diagrams and a 3D skull model from the anatomy lab. Aligning the model with the illustrations allowed me to visualize the sinus's location in relation to surrounding structures like the nasal cavity and zygomatic bone.

One memorable study session involved using a flashlight to shine through the model, simulating the function of the sinus. This interactive technique clarified my understanding and made the learning process memorable. By incorporating physical models alongside visual aids, I could better grasp the anatomy in a clinical context, reinforcing the information for future application.

5. Creating Personal Associations: Connecting with Your Studies

Creating personal associations can also enhance memorization. While studying the dental nerves, I linked each nerve to a personal memory or story. For example, I connected the Inferior Alveolar Nerve to my childhood experience of getting braces. This connection made the nerve's clinical relevance much clearer and easier to remember.

By weaving my personal experiences into my studies, I transformed abstract concepts into relatable narratives, making them easier to recall during exams. This strategy not only reinforced my memory but also made studying feel more meaningful and connected to my life.

6. Creating a Single Word from a List of Terms

A fun and effective technique I utilized involved creating single words from lists of terms. For example, if I had to memorize the different types of teeth (incisors, canines, premolars, molars), I combined the first letters of each type to create a memorable acronym: I.C.P.M. I visualized a whimsical character, "I.C. the Tooth Fairy," who would remind me of each tooth type. This approach made recalling the list easier, as I could simply think of the acronym and its associated character to trigger my memory.

Memorizing dental anatomy doesn't have to be an arduous task. By embracing visual mnemonics, rhythmic techniques, hands-on learning, personal associations, and creative wordplay, you can transform your study sessions into engaging experiences that foster deeper understanding and retention. These strategies not only aid in memorization but also make learning enjoyable, ensuring that the knowledge you gain during your dental studies will stay with you throughout your career. So, embrace these techniques, get creative, and watch your confidence grow as you master the art and science of dentistry!

Utilizing Visual Learning Tools: Mind Mapping

As dental students, we often grapple with intricate concepts that can be overwhelming, particularly in demanding subjects like pharmacology and pathology. One transformative strategy that has significantly enhanced my understanding and retention of this complex information is the use of visual learning tools, especially mind mapping. This technique not only streamlines the learning process but also makes it far more enjoyable.

What is Mind Mapping?

Mind mapping is a visual representation of information that allows you to organize and connect concepts in a hierarchical manner. It begins with a central idea, from which branches extend to related topics and subtopics. This method caters to visual learners and is especially helpful in subjects that require understanding the relationships between various elements, such as drug classifications and pathological processes.

The beauty of mind mapping lies in its ability to turn dense blocks of text into a vibrant visual representation, helping to clarify complex ideas and enhance recall. It's about transforming abstract concepts into a concrete, visual format that your brain can easily navigate.

Creating Effective Mind Maps

When I first started using mind maps, I focused on breaking down the vast amount of information in pharmacology into manageable parts. For example, I would label my central node "Pharmacology." From there, I would draw branches for each drug category—like analgesics, antibiotics, and antihypertensives—linking these branches to specific drugs, their mechanisms of action, side effects, and clinical applications.

On one particularly memorable evening, as I prepared for a pharmacology exam, I decided to create an extensive mind map sprawled out on my living room floor. Armed with large sheets of paper and colorful markers, I drew my central node and watched my ideas blossom outward like a web. Each branch was a new opportunity to explore connections: I could visually relate how beta-blockers functioned as antihypertensives and how different antibiotic classes acted against bacterial mechanisms. This visual representation transformed my review sessions from monotonous note-flipping into an engaging exploration of the material.

Enhancing Retention Through Visualization

One of the most rewarding aspects of mind mapping is how it fosters an exhilarating sense of connection between concepts. As I moved from one branch to another, the relationships between drugs and their applications became clearer, reinforcing my understanding in a way that rote memorization simply could not achieve. For instance, while mapping out the side effects of various medications, I could visually relate these to their pharmacological actions, which helped me remember why certain drugs had specific side effects.

Incorporating color-coding into my mind maps took this experience to another level. I used different colored pens to distinguish between categories, such as green for antibiotics, blue for analgesics, and red for side effects. This not only made the mind maps visually appealing but also enhanced their effectiveness as study tools. During review sessions, the colors helped my brain quickly identify related concepts, allowing me to digest the information more efficiently.

Collaborative Mind Mapping

Mind mapping also serves as an excellent collaborative tool. I frequently studied with classmates, and together, we would create mind maps that integrated our insights and perspectives. During one particularly fruitful group study session, we tackled the topic of cardiac drugs. Each of us contributed to the mind map by adding our understanding of how different medications impacted heart function, their indications, and contraindications. This collaborative effort not only expanded our collective knowledge but also fostered a sense of community among us as we navigated the complexities of pharmacology together.

By pooling our resources and engaging in discussions around the mind map, we were able to see various perspectives on the same topic, which deepened our understanding and retention. The act of teaching one another solidified our learning, demonstrating the power of collaboration in the educational process.

Practical Application and Reflection

The benefits of mind mapping extend beyond exam preparation; I've found it incredibly useful during clinical rotations. In practice, understanding the pathophysiology of conditions and their treatments is crucial. For instance, when I encountered a patient with diabetes, I would quickly sketch a mind map in my notes to visualize the relationship between different types of insulin, their actions, and the corresponding patient management strategies. This approach allowed me to apply theoretical knowledge to practical scenarios, reinforcing my learning and enhancing my confidence in patient care.

I vividly recall an afternoon in the clinic where I had to explain diabetes management to a patient. Having recently created a mind map summarizing insulin types, their actions, and the monitoring protocols, I felt equipped to provide a clear and informed explanation. The visualization helped me connect the dots in real-time, ensuring that I communicated the information effectively.

Incorporating mind mapping into your study routine can profoundly impact your learning experience in dental school. This visual tool not only aids in organizing complex information but also enhances your ability to see connections between concepts, making the material more relatable and easier to recall. By creating vibrant, dynamic mind maps, you engage with the content on a deeper level, leading to a more comprehensive understanding of pharmacology, pathology, and beyond.

So, gather your colored pens and large sheets of paper, and start mapping out your thoughts. As you transform your study sessions into visual explorations, you'll likely discover newfound enthusiasm and clarity in your learning journey. Mind mapping is not just a study tool; it's an engaging and interactive way to navigate the intricate world of dentistry, paving the way for both academic success and clinical excellence. By embracing this technique, you'll empower yourself to tackle the challenges of dental school with confidence and creativity.

The Feynman Technique in Dental Studies: A Practical Approach

The Feynman Technique is a powerful learning tool that helps break down complex topics by focusing on simplicity and clarity. Named after Nobel Prize-winning physicist Richard Feynman, this method encourages you to explain a topic in your own words as if you were teaching it to someone with no background knowledge on the subject. In dental studies, where dense and technical information can be overwhelming, the Feynman Technique can be a highly effective way to build understanding and retention. Here's how you can apply it to specific dental subjects:

Step 1: Choose a Concept You Want to Learn

Begin with a specific dental topic you're studying. Let's say you want to master the concept of tooth development stages or understand the periodontal ligament and its role in oral health. These subjects involve a lot of technical terms, but the Feynman Technique can help make sense of them.

Step 2: Explain the Concept in Simple Terms

Here's where the Feynman Technique's magic happens. Try to explain the concept as if you were teaching it to someone new to dentistry—perhaps a friend or even a child. For example:

Tooth Development Stages: "Teeth don't just appear fully formed in the mouth; they go through a series of stages to grow.

First, there's a 'bud stage,' where the cells start forming the basic shape. Next, we have a 'cap stage,' where more layers form around this bud, making it look like a tiny cap. Eventually, in the 'bell stage,' it starts looking like a tooth with enamel and dentin. By the time it erupts, the tooth has grown its crown and is getting ready to emerge in the mouth."

Explaining in simple language helps ensure you understand each part rather than memorizing it.

Step 3: Identify Gaps in Your Knowledge

While explaining, you may stumble or realize certain areas aren't clear. This is a key part of the Feynman Technique because it shows you what you don't fully understand. For instance, you may realize you're unsure how exactly enamel forms during the bell stage or what happens in the cap stage that's critical for dental health.

In such cases, revisit your textbook or lecture notes and clarify these points. Look up information in other resources, such as illustrations, diagrams, or even YouTube videos. This reinforces your understanding and helps fill in the gaps.

Step 4: Simplify Further Using Analogies or Visual Aids

Once you've clarified the concept, refine it even more by using analogies or visual aids. Here are some ways you might do this:

Tooth Development Stages Analogy: Compare tooth development to the growth of a tree. The bud stage is like a tree seedling starting to sprout, the cap stage is when branches form, and the bell stage is the tree maturing and growing strong roots and branches.

Periodontal Ligament: The periodontal ligament, which connects the tooth to the jaw, can be compared to the ropes on a suspension bridge. Just as ropes stabilize the bridge while allowing slight movement, the periodontal ligament supports the tooth and absorbs forces when we chew, while also allowing tiny movements.

These analogies help you visualize and remember complex concepts in a simple way.

Step 5: Review and Summarize

To reinforce what you've learned, try summarizing the topic in a few sentences, focusing on the core aspects. Here's an example of a summary:

Tooth Development Summary: "Tooth development happens in three main stages: the bud stage (basic tooth shape formation), the cap stage (formation of layers around the tooth bud), and the bell stage (formation of enamel and dentin). By the end of these stages, the tooth is ready to erupt in the mouth with its crown fully developed."

Or for Periodontal Ligament: Periodontal Ligament Summary: "The periodontal ligament is a connective tissue that attaches the tooth to the jawbone. It acts as a shock absorber, protecting the tooth from strong chewing forces and allowing tiny, protective movements."

Revisiting your notes or re-explaining the concept every few days also helps retain it long-term.

Example Application to Other Dental Subjects

1. Anatomy of the Temporomandibular Joint (TMJ):

Explanation: The TMJ is like a hinge that allows your jaw to open and close, and it has a small disk between the bones to prevent grinding.

 Gaps Identified: While explaining, you might notice you're unsure about the specific muscles involved in jaw movement.

Analogy: Compare the TMJ to a door hinge with a cushion inside, allowing the door (jaw) to move smoothly.

Summary: "The TMJ connects the jaw to the skull, has a protective disk, and enables movements essential for chewing and speaking."

2. Dental Caries Development and Prevention:

Explanation: Dental caries is the breakdown of tooth enamel caused by bacteria producing acids from sugar. It's like when acid corrodes metal, breaking down the surface over time.

Gaps Identified: You might discover you're unclear about the exact process of demineralization and remineralization.

Analogy: Compare enamel to a castle wall that bacteria attack with acid like a battering ram.

Summary: "Dental caries forms when bacteria break down sugars into acids, which erode tooth enamel. Fluoride can help repair these tiny damages and strengthen the enamel."

By using the Feynman Technique, you're not only learning concepts for an exam but also developing a deep, practical understanding that will be invaluable in clinical practice. This approach can make complex dental subjects more approachable, strengthen your teaching skills, and ultimately improve your confidence as a future dentist.

The SQ3R Method for Effective Reading

In the whirlwind of dental school, where every moment is precious and the volume of information can feel overwhelming, mastering effective reading strategies is essential. One technique that has significantly enhanced my comprehension and retention of complex material is the SQ3R method—Survey, Question, Read, Recite, and Review. This structured approach to reading transforms passive skimming into an active learning process, making it a game-changer for any dental student.

Understanding the SQ3R Method

The SQ3R method is designed to help you engage with your reading material more deeply and effectively. Each step of the process builds upon the last, creating a comprehensive framework that enhances both understanding and memory retention. Here's how it works in detail:

1. Survey: The first step involves quickly skimming the chapter. Before diving into the dense text, I take a few moments to scan the headings, subheadings, and any visuals such as diagrams or charts. This provides a roadmap of what to expect. For example, while preparing for a chapter on oral microbiology, I might notice headings that outline key topics like "Normal Flora," "Pathogenic Bacteria," and "Antimicrobial Therapy." This initial survey helps me grasp the scope of the chapter and sets the stage for deeper exploration.

2. Question: Next, I transform the headings into questions to guide my reading. This step is crucial as it creates a purpose for my study. Continuing with the oral microbiology chapter, I would formulate questions like, "What are the key bacteria found in the oral cavity?" and "How do these bacteria interact with the host?" By establishing questions, I prime my brain to look for answers as I read, enhancing focus and engagement. This not only keeps me on track but also turns the reading experience into an active quest for knowledge.

3. Read: With my questions in mind, I dive into the reading. This is where I take my time to thoroughly absorb the material. I highlight key points and make notes in the margins, especially when I come across information that answers my earlier questions. For instance, while reading about Streptococcus mutans, I would note its role in dental caries formation and its ability to produce acid, emphasizing how it contributes to tooth decay. This active reading not only aids comprehension but also makes the material feel more personal and relevant to my studies.

4. Recite: After finishing a section, I close the book and recite what I've learned in my own words. This step is vital for reinforcing memory retention. By verbalizing the material, I actively engage with it. For example, I might summarize that "Streptococcus mutans is a significant contributor to dental caries due to its acidogenic properties." This practice not only solidifies the information but also helps identify any gaps in my understanding that I may need to revisit. I find that this act of recitation transforms information from a passive experience into a dynamic conversation with myself, making the knowledge more tangible.

5. Review: The final step involves revisiting my notes or mind maps to reinforce the material. I find that reviewing my summaries and mind maps after completing a chapter helps cement the information in my memory. It's a way to connect the dots between different concepts, such as linking the pathogenic bacteria discussed to their clinical implications in dentistry. By setting aside time at the end of each week to review, I ensure that the material remains fresh in my mind, preparing me for exams and practical applications.

Transforming My Study Sessions

Implementing the SQ3R method revolutionized my reading sessions from passive tasks into active learning experiences. I vividly remember preparing for a particularly challenging exam on dental materials. Before adopting SQ3R, I often felt overwhelmed by the volume of information and struggled to recall specifics during exams. However, by using this method, I transformed my reading into an engaging process. I was not just skimming text; I was actively seeking answers and constructing my understanding.

As I prepared, I could recall the properties of different dental materials, their applications, and their implications in practice with greater ease. For instance, while studying composites, I generated questions like, "What are the benefits of using composite materials for restorations?" As I read, I highlighted important characteristics such as their aesthetic advantages and versatility in various clinical situations. The structured approach gave me the confidence I needed walking into the exam room. I remember feeling a surge of reassurance as I recognized key concepts—thanks to the questions I had generated earlier and the summaries I had recited.

The SQ3R method is more than just a reading strategy; it's a powerful tool that can enhance your learning experience in dental school. By transforming the way you approach reading—turning it into an active and engaging process—you'll find that you retain information better and feel more prepared for exams. This method encourages critical thinking, fosters deeper understanding, and ultimately equips you with the tools you need to succeed in your dental education.

So, the next time you sit down with your textbooks, give the SQ3R method a try. Approach your readings with curiosity and purpose, and watch as your comprehension and retention soar. This simple yet effective strategy can make a significant difference in your academic journey, paving the way for both understanding and confidence in your future practice as a dental professional.

Collaborative Study vs. Individual Study: Finding Your Balance

In the demanding environment of dental school, where every moment is precious and the volume of material can be overwhelming, finding the right study approach is essential for success. As you navigate this complex landscape, discovering a balance between collaborative study and individual study can significantly enhance your learning experience and overall well-being.

The Benefits of Collaborative Study

Collaborative study sessions are an invaluable resource for dental students. They foster motivation, accountability, and diverse perspectives that can deepen your understanding of complex topics. When studying in groups, you benefit from the varied strengths and knowledge of your peers. For instance, during a group session focused on dental materials, we would each take turns explaining our favorite materials. Some classmates discussed the properties and applications of composite resins, while others delved into the intricacies of glass ionomers. This collective sharing not only solidified my own understanding but also introduced me to concepts and applications I might not have encountered studying alone.

Moreover, collaborating with others can expose you to innovative ideas and real-world applications. One memorable session revolved around periodontal disease. As each member of our group took on a different aspect of the topic—one focusing on diagnosis, another discussing treatment options, and a third presenting case studies—we collectively pieced together a comprehensive understanding of the condition. One of my classmates even shared a recent case from their clinical experiences that highlighted an innovative treatment approach. Hearing these real-world applications helped solidify my understanding and encouraged me to think critically about treatment options.

To maximize the effectiveness of these group sessions, it's crucial to set clear goals for each meeting. For example, we might decide that one session would be dedicated to mastering the intricacies of dental anatomy, while another would tackle pharmacology concepts. This structured approach ensured that our time together was productive and targeted, allowing us to delve deeply into each subject area without straying off course.

The Value of Individual Study

While group study offers numerous benefits, individual study time is equally important. Solo study allows for deep focus on your unique learning needs and preferences. I often reserved quiet time for reflection and concentrated study, especially when I needed to master intricate details or tackle challenging concepts. For example, when preparing for an exam on oral pathology, I would isolate myself in the library with my notes and textbooks, allowing me to absorb the material without distractions. This deep dive was essential for topics that required synthesizing information, such as understanding the differences between various oral lesions and their clinical implications.

I discovered that some topics required more individual attention than others. For instance, while group discussions on anatomy were beneficial, I needed extra hours alone to use models and diagrams to visualize structures thoroughly. This personalized approach allowed me to master challenging concepts at my own pace without the pressure of keeping up with others, ensuring that I was well-prepared for practical applications in the clinic.

Striking the Right Balance

Finding the right balance between collaborative and individual study is essential for maximizing your effectiveness as a dental student. I often alternated between the two approaches, ensuring I harnessed the strengths of each. One effective strategy was to use group study sessions for discussion and reinforcement while reserving quiet time for deeper reflection and concentrated study.

To maximize our group sessions, we would come prepared with specific topics to focus on, whether it was dental materials or the principles of endodontics. This not only kept our discussions organized but also allowed us to build on each other's knowledge. I remember a particularly impactful session where we all presented on different aspects of periodontal disease. Each member shared their findings on diagnosis, treatment options, and relevant case studies, reinforcing our learning and fostering a sense of teamwork.

Additionally, the camaraderie built during these study sessions made the experience more enjoyable and less isolating. Knowing that I had a supportive network to lean on during challenging times proved invaluable, especially as we approached finals. Sharing personal experiences and stress management techniques during our meetings transformed our study group into a source of encouragement and motivation.

In conclusion, finding the right balance between collaborative study and individual study is crucial for success in dental school. Both methods offer unique advantages that, when combined, create a more enriching learning experience. Collaborative study fosters motivation, accountability, and diverse perspectives, while individual study allows for deep focus and personalized understanding.

As you navigate your dental education, I encourage you to embrace both collaborative and individual study methods. Experiment with different strategies to find what works best for you, and don't underestimate the power of working together with your peers. This balance will not only help you master the material but also build lasting relationships that can support you throughout your career. Ultimately, striking this equilibrium between collaboration and solitude can enhance your understanding and retention of complex material, preparing you for a successful and fulfilling career in dentistry.

Mastering effective study techniques in dental school isn't merely about working harder; it's about working smarter. By incorporating active learning, utilizing memory strategies, managing your time effectively, and leveraging visual tools, you'll find that not only does the material become easier to understand, but your confidence will also grow.

Remember, dental school is a journey filled with challenges, but each step you take toward mastering these techniques lays the foundation for your future as a skilled dental professional. Embrace the challenges, foster connections with your peers, and savor the process of learning. Your future as a competent and compassionate dentist awaits, ready to make a significant impact in the lives of your patients. So, take a deep breath, dive into your studies, and enjoy the adventure ahead!

Time Management and Work-Life Balance

Time management and work-life balance are crucial skills to master as a dental student, especially given the rigorous demands of dental education. Juggling study schedules, clinical responsibilities, and personal life can feel overwhelming at times, but creating a realistic routine that incorporates moments of self-care and socialization is essential for maintaining both your mental health and academic performance.

Strategies for Effective Time Management

1. Prioritize Tasks: Start each day by listing your tasks in order of priority. Identify what absolutely needs to be accomplished that day and what can wait. This clarity will help you avoid feeling overwhelmed.

2. Use a Planner: Whether it's a digital calendar or a physical planner, keeping track of deadlines, classes, and social events can help you visualize your time and manage it more effectively.

3. Set Specific Study Times: Designate specific blocks of time for studying. This helps to create a routine and builds discipline. Make sure to stick to these times as closely as possible to form a habit.

4. Incorporate Breaks: Use techniques like the Pomodoro Technique—study for 25 minutes, then take a 5-minute break. This not only helps maintain focus but also allows your brain to recharge.

5. Schedule Social Activities: Just as you schedule study sessions, plan social activities. This could be a weekly dinner with friends, a movie night, or even a short walk in the park. Knowing you have something to look forward to can motivate you to stay focused during your study times.

6. Practice Self-Care: Set aside time for self-care activities that help you relax and recharge. Whether it's reading, exercising, meditating, or pursuing a hobby, these moments are crucial for maintaining your mental health.

Embracing Flexibility

Another key element of time management is the ability to remain flexible. Life can be unpredictable, and sometimes your plans will change. Perhaps you need to reschedule study time because of a family obligation or a sudden illness. Embrace these changes with an open mind. Adaptability is a skill that will serve you well in both your personal life and your future dental practice.

The Long-Term Perspective

Remember, dental school is just one phase of your life. It's important to cultivate a holistic view of your well-being that includes academic success, personal happiness, and meaningful relationships. The habits you develop now will shape your future practice and approach to patient care. A dentist who knows how to balance their time effectively is likely to bring that same care and balance into their interactions with patients, creating a more positive experience for everyone involved.

Ultimately, mastering time management and work-life balance in dental school is about more than just getting through exams. It's about preparing yourself for a fulfilling career where you can excel professionally while also enjoying a rich and rewarding personal life. Embrace your studies, but don't forget to live. Celebrate small victories, find joy in friendships, and create memories that will sustain you through the challenges of dental education and beyond. Balancing work and play may not always be easy, but it's a skill worth developing for the sake of your future, your patients, and yourself.

Utilizing Technology for Studying

In today's educational landscape, technology serves as an invaluable ally for students, especially in a demanding field like dentistry. Embracing digital resources not only enhances your learning experience but also helps simplify complex concepts that can often feel overwhelming. Let me share my journey of how technology transformed my studying habits and led to deeper understanding and better retention of information.

The Power of Online Resources

I vividly recall a particular moment during my first year when I was struggling to grasp the intricacies of dental anatomy. The textbook definitions were dense and full of jargon that felt alien to me. One evening, while feeling frustrated and stuck, I stumbled upon an online video that broke down the topic into clear, digestible pieces.

The presenter used engaging visuals and simplified language to explain each structure, which made it feel like a conversation rather than a lecture. It was as if a light bulb had suddenly illuminated my mind. Concepts that once seemed convoluted transformed into something relatable and understandable. This experience taught me the power of diverse learning methods and how a single video could make a significant difference in my comprehension.

Embracing Various Technologies

1. Online Tutorials and Videos: As I continued my studies, I discovered an array of online platforms dedicated to dental education. Websites like YouTube, Coursera, and Khan Academy offer a wealth of tutorials on everything from basic concepts to advanced procedures. Whenever I faced a difficult topic, I would search for video explanations. These visual aids allowed me to see concepts in action, whether it was a demonstration of a dental procedure or an animation illustrating the anatomy of the oral cavity.

2. Educational Apps: There are numerous apps specifically designed for dental students. For instance, apps like "Dentistry 101" and "Dental Anatomy" feature interactive diagrams and quizzes that engage you in active learning. I found it incredibly helpful to use these apps for quick reviews between classes or during breaks. The gamified quizzes turned study sessions into fun challenges rather than tedious tasks.

3. Interactive Study Platforms: Platforms like Quizlet and Anki revolutionized my memorization techniques. By creating flashcards for important terms and concepts, I was able to study effectively and efficiently. The spaced repetition feature in these apps ensured that I revisited difficult material at optimal intervals, reinforcing my memory over time. I remember the satisfaction of gradually mastering topics that initially intimidated me, all thanks to this interactive approach.

4. ChatGPT and AI Assistance: One of the most game-changing tools in my study arsenal became AI-driven platforms like ChatGPT. Whenever I had questions that arose during my studies, I would turn to these platforms for clarification. For example, if I was unsure about the steps in a specific procedure or needed a breakdown of a complex topic, I would type out my questions. The responses I received were often more concise and tailored to my level of understanding than traditional sources. This interaction felt almost like having a personal tutor available 24/7, ready to assist whenever I needed help.

Collaborative Learning Through Technology

Another aspect of utilizing technology is the ability to collaborate with peers. During group study sessions, we often relied on shared digital tools like Google Docs or online whiteboards to brainstorm ideas and compile notes. These collaborative platforms made it easy to divide topics among us and create comprehensive study materials that we could all access.

I remember one late-night study session where we were preparing for an upcoming exam on periodontology. Using a shared Google Slide presentation, we divided the topics and each created slides summarizing key points, visuals, and even quiz questions. This not only made studying more engaging but also helped us learn from each other's perspectives and insights. When we later quizzed each other using the slides, it solidified our understanding and made studying feel more like a team effort rather than a solitary task.

Balancing Technology and Traditional Methods

While technology is a powerful resource, it's important to strike a balance between digital and traditional study methods. For example, while I loved using apps and videos, I also made it a point to incorporate physical textbooks and handwritten notes into my routine. There's something about the tactile experience of writing things down that aids retention and helps you internalize information.

Additionally, during clinical practice, while I relied on digital resources for theoretical knowledge, I made sure to apply what I learned in real-life scenarios. Observing procedures, practicing techniques on models, and engaging with patients helped bridge the gap between virtual learning and practical application.

Utilizing technology in your studies is not just about finding shortcuts; it's about enhancing your understanding and creating a more dynamic learning experience. The online videos, educational apps, interactive platforms, and AI tools all played a crucial role in my journey through dental school. They made complex concepts accessible, fostered collaborative learning, and helped me stay engaged in my studies.

As you embark on your own educational journey, I encourage you to explore the plethora of technological resources available to you. Embrace them as partners in your learning process, and don't be afraid to experiment with different tools to discover what works best for you. By leveraging technology effectively, you can transform your study habits, boost your confidence, and pave the way for a successful career in dentistry.

Final Thoughts

In conclusion, building a solid study foundation in dental school is an art that combines effective study techniques, time management, and the ability to maintain a work-life balance. By utilizing active learning strategies and engaging with your peers, you'll not only improve your retention of complex material but also foster a supportive community that will help you thrive. Remember, as you delve into the fascinating world of dentistry, it's not just about memorizing facts; it's about internalizing knowledge and applying it with skill and compassion. Embrace the journey, learn from every experience, and enjoy the ride—it's a path that will lead to both personal and professional fulfillment.

Chapter 3 - Mastering Dental-Specific Study Techniques

As you navigate through the complexities of dental courses, especially anatomy, pharmacology, and dental materials, unique memorization strategies will become your best friends. Visual learning through diagrams and models can make the dense material more digestible. Hands-on skills are equally important; practicing your hand-eye coordination and spatial awareness outside the lab can greatly enhance your confidence when it's time to work on real patients. I remember spending hours at home, practicing my dexterity with simple tools, mimicking the movements I would need in the clinic. As the saying goes, "Practice makes perfect," and I found this to be particularly true.

Tricks and Techniques for Studying Anatomy of Head and Neck

Studying the anatomy of the head and neck can be one of the most intricate yet rewarding parts of dental education. The complexity of structures, from muscles and nerves to blood vessels and bones, requires an effective approach to make sense of it all. Below are some tricks and techniques I found invaluable during my studies, each designed to enhance understanding and retention of this vital subject.

1. Use of Visual Aids

Anatomy is inherently a visual subject, so utilizing diagrams, models, and 3D anatomy apps can significantly enhance your learning experience. I found that traditional textbooks often failed to provide a clear picture of spatial relationships. Instead, I invested in a high-quality anatomy atlas that offered detailed images and descriptions. One particular atlas featured cross-sectional views, which helped me visualize how structures relate to each other in three dimensions.

In addition to static images, interactive 3D apps like "Complete Anatomy" or "Visible Body" allowed me to manipulate models, isolating specific structures to see how they fit together. For instance, when studying the muscles of mastication, I could rotate the model to see how the masseter and temporalis muscles interacted during jaw movements, which deepened my understanding of functional anatomy.

2. Drawing and Labeling

Engaging with the material actively through drawing can solidify your knowledge. I would often spend time sketching key structures, such as the cranial nerves or the vascular supply to the head and neck, labeling each part as I went. This method not only reinforced my memory but also helped me recognize connections between different anatomical features.

For example, while drawing the arterial supply of the head, I made a comprehensive diagram that included the common carotid artery, its bifurcation into the internal and external carotid arteries, and the branches supplying the face and scalp. Each label was accompanied by notes on the functions and clinical relevance of each artery, which proved invaluable for my exams and later clinical practice.

3. Mnemonics and Memory Aids

Creating mnemonics can be a game-changer when trying to remember complex anatomical information. For cranial nerves, I found it helpful to use phrases that were both memorable and relevant. For instance, to recall the order of the twelve cranial nerves, I used the phrase: "Oh, Oh, Oh, To Touch And Feel Very Green Vegetables, AH!" Each initial corresponds to a cranial nerve. This simple trick allowed me to quickly recall the names and order of the nerves during both exams and clinical situations.

Additionally, associating structures with vivid imagery can enhance recall. For instance, when learning about the facial nerve's path, I imagined it as a performer gracefully moving across the stage of the face, innervating muscles as it went. Such mental imagery made the learning process more engaging and memorable.

4. Group Study Sessions

Studying anatomy with classmates can provide different perspectives and explanations that clarify challenging concepts. During my time in dental school, I participated in group study sessions where we would quiz each other on different topics. For example, one week, we focused on the muscles of the neck. Each member prepared a short presentation on a specific muscle, including its origin, insertion, function, and innervation.

One of my classmates created a physical model using clay to demonstrate the muscles, which provided a tangible reference that made the information more relatable. This collaborative effort not only reinforced our individual understanding but also fostered a sense of camaraderie, which made studying less stressful.

5. Clinical Correlation

Integrating clinical relevance into your studies can significantly enhance your understanding of anatomical structures. Whenever I learned about a particular nerve or vessel, I sought to understand its clinical implications. For instance, when studying the trigeminal nerve, I researched its role in dental anesthesia and the clinical significance of its branches.

By understanding how the maxillary and mandibular branches of the trigeminal nerve are anesthetized during dental procedures, I could connect the theoretical knowledge to practical applications. This approach not only made studying more interesting but also equipped me with the knowledge I would need in the clinic.

6. Regular Review and Self-Testing

Anatomy requires consistent review due to its vast amount of information. I established a routine where I would dedicate a portion of my study time each week to revisiting previously covered material. Utilizing flashcards, I created a set for the bones of the skull, labeling each part and its features.

I would test myself regularly, quizzing myself on the functions of different nerves and their pathways. This spaced repetition reinforced my memory and helped keep the information fresh in my mind, making it easier to recall during exams and clinical scenarios.

Mastering the anatomy of the head and neck is a formidable task, but employing a variety of tricks and techniques can make the process not only manageable but also enjoyable. By using visual aids, engaging in active drawing, employing mnemonics, collaborating with peers, integrating clinical relevance, and committing to regular review, you can build a solid foundation in head and neck anatomy.

As you progress through your studies, remember to be patient with yourself and to find strategies that resonate with your learning style. The knowledge you gain in this area will be essential in your journey as a dental professional, impacting both your clinical skills and your ability to provide the best care for your patients. Embrace the challenge, and you'll find that your efforts will pay off in ways that enhance both your education and your future career.

Tricks and Techniques for Studying Human Physiology in Dental School

Studying human physiology is a critical component of dental education, as it provides the foundational understanding of how the body functions—essential knowledge for any aspiring dentist. The intricate systems of the body and their interconnections can be overwhelming, but with the right techniques and tricks, you can make your study of human physiology both effective and engaging. Here are some strategies that can help you navigate this complex subject with confidence.

1. Utilize Active Learning Techniques

One of the most effective ways to grasp complex physiological concepts is through active learning. This approach involves engaging directly with the material rather than passively reading or listening. Techniques such as teaching others, creating flashcards, or working on practice questions can be immensely beneficial.

For example, after learning about the cardiovascular system, I would explain the flow of blood through the heart and major vessels to a study partner. Teaching someone else forces you to clarify your understanding and address any gaps in your knowledge. Flashcards can also be handy for memorizing key terms and definitions, such as the differences between systolic and diastolic pressures, or the roles of various neurotransmitters. Utilizing spaced repetition when reviewing flashcards can enhance retention, as you revisit the information at increasing intervals.

2. Visualize Complex Processes

Human physiology often involves dynamic processes that are easier to understand when visualized. Diagrams, flowcharts, and videos can transform complex information into more digestible formats. For instance, when studying the nephron's role in kidney function, I found it helpful to draw a detailed diagram of the nephron, labeling each part and its function. This visual representation helped me see how blood filtration and urine formation occurred, reinforcing my understanding of the material.

Additionally, educational platforms like YouTube offer a wealth of visual resources. I often turned to channels that provided animations of physiological processes, such as muscle contraction or synaptic transmission. These animations can make the mechanisms behind these processes more tangible and easier to remember.

3. Make Connections Between Topics

Physiology does not exist in isolation; it's intertwined with various aspects of biology and dentistry. Creating connections between topics can enhance comprehension and retention. For example, when studying the respiratory system, I made it a point to relate it to the dental field by exploring how respiratory health can affect oral health—such as the impact of mouth breathing on dental alignment and gum health.

I also kept a running list of "connections" in a notebook, where I noted how different systems interacted, like how the endocrine system influences metabolic processes that can impact dental treatments. This integrative approach not only enriched my understanding but also made the learning experience more meaningful.

4. Practice Clinical Applications

Applying your knowledge to clinical scenarios is a great way to solidify your understanding of physiology. During our courses, we often discussed case studies that illustrated how physiological principles applied to patient care. For example, when learning about the autonomic nervous system, we analyzed a case where a patient presented with hypertension. Understanding how the sympathetic and parasympathetic systems influenced heart rate and vascular resistance helped us think critically about potential treatments.

I also utilized practice questions from textbooks or online resources that posed clinical scenarios, which challenged me to apply what I had learned. This technique not only prepared me for exams but also reinforced the real-world relevance of the material.

5. Create a Study Schedule

With the extensive content covered in human physiology, it's essential to create a structured study schedule that allows you to break down the material into manageable sections. Instead of cramming, I often planned my study sessions around specific topics. For instance, I would allocate one week to the nervous system, focusing on its structure and function each day.

Using techniques like the Pomodoro Technique, I set timers for focused study intervals followed by short breaks. This method kept me engaged without feeling overwhelmed, and I found it particularly effective for absorbing dense material.

6. Join or Form Study Groups

Collaboration can significantly enhance your understanding of human physiology. Joining or forming a study group with your classmates can provide diverse perspectives and insights. In my own experience, our study group would meet weekly to tackle challenging topics. For example, we dissected the complexities of the gastrointestinal system by assigning each member a segment to research and present.

This collaborative effort not only helped us share the workload but also provided a platform for discussion, where we could ask questions and clarify doubts. The social aspect of studying together also made the process more enjoyable and less isolating.

7. Stay Curious and Ask Questions

Lastly, fostering a mindset of curiosity can transform your study of human physiology. Don't hesitate to ask questions in class or during group discussions. I remember being intrigued by the endocrine system's role in metabolism and how it influenced dental health. My curiosity prompted me to approach my professor after class, leading to a deeper conversation that further enriched my understanding.

Keeping a journal of questions as you study can help you stay engaged and encourage you to explore topics more thoroughly. This habit not only enhances your learning but also prepares you for a career in dentistry, where curiosity and inquiry are essential traits.

Studying human physiology can be a challenging yet rewarding journey in dental school. By employing active learning techniques, visualizing complex processes, making connections, practicing clinical applications, organizing your study time, collaborating with peers, and fostering a curious mindset, you can enhance your understanding and retention of this vital subject. Remember that mastering physiology is not just about passing exams; it's about laying the groundwork for a successful career in dentistry, where this knowledge will inform your clinical decisions and patient care. Embrace the process, and don't hesitate to seek support from your peers and instructors along the way.

Tricks and Techniques for Studying Biochemistry in Dental School

Biochemistry can often feel like a daunting subject for dental students, intertwining complex molecular concepts with the biological functions relevant to our future practices. However, with the right strategies and techniques, you can turn biochemistry into a manageable and even enjoyable part of your studies. Here are some effective tricks and techniques that can help you master this crucial subject.

1. Visual Learning: Diagrams and Flowcharts

Biochemistry is a visual subject; it thrives on understanding the relationships between different molecules and processes. One of the most effective techniques I found was to create detailed diagrams and flowcharts. For instance, when studying metabolic pathways such as glycolysis or the citric acid cycle, I would map out each step, noting key enzymes, substrates, and products.

By visualizing these pathways, I could see how they interconnected, which helped me grasp the bigger picture. I also found it beneficial to color-code these diagrams based on categories, such as reactants, products, and enzymes. This not only made the diagrams more engaging but also helped reinforce memory through visual associations.

2. Mnemonic Devices: Memory Aids

Another powerful tool for tackling biochemistry is the use of mnemonic devices. The field is filled with complex terms and sequences that can be challenging to memorize. For instance, when studying the essential amino acids, I used the mnemonic "Private Tim Hall" to remember: P (Phenylalanine), T (Threonine), I (Isoleucine), M (Methionine), H (Histidine), A (Arginine), L (Leucine), L (Lysine).

This technique not only made memorization easier but also injected a bit of fun into my study sessions. Creating your own mnemonics can be particularly effective, as personalizing them helps embed the information in your memory.

3. Active Recall and Spaced Repetition

Active recall is a learning strategy that involves retrieving information from memory rather than passively reviewing notes. To implement this, I would frequently test myself on the material. For example, after studying enzyme kinetics, I would write down everything I remembered about Michaelis-Menten kinetics, including the equation and what each variable represented.

In conjunction with active recall, I used spaced repetition software (like Anki) to revisit these concepts at increasing intervals. This combination solidified my understanding and helped keep the information fresh in my mind leading up to exams.

4. Application Through Case Studies

Understanding the clinical relevance of biochemistry can greatly enhance your retention and motivation. Whenever I encountered a new concept, such as the role of enzymes in digestion, I would look for clinical case studies or examples that illustrated these processes in a real-world context.

For instance, learning about the deficiency of certain enzymes, like lactase in lactose intolerance, allowed me to connect the biochemical concepts to actual patient scenarios. This approach not only made the material more engaging but also reinforced my understanding of how biochemistry applies directly to dentistry and patient care.

5. Study Groups and Collaborative Learning

Biochemistry is a subject where discussing concepts with peers can significantly enhance your understanding. Forming study groups provided a platform for sharing insights and tackling complex topics collaboratively. In one memorable study session, we focused on biochemical signalling pathways. Each member was assigned a different pathway to research and present, such as the insulin signalling pathway or the GPCR pathway.

This method not only diversified our learning but also highlighted the interconnectedness of various pathways and their implications in health and disease. The discussions that followed each presentation deepened our collective understanding and often led to illuminating questions and insights that I might not have considered on my own.

6. Utilizing Online Resources and Apps

In today's digital age, numerous online resources can enhance your biochemistry studies. Websites like Khan Academy, YouTube, and various mobile apps offer tutorials, animations, and quizzes that cater to different learning styles. I found that watching animated videos explaining complex processes, such as protein synthesis or metabolic regulation, made it easier to grasp these concepts visually.

Moreover, many biochemistry textbooks come with online access codes that provide additional resources such as practice quizzes and interactive flashcards. Engaging with these tools can supplement your study routine and help reinforce your understanding.

7. Integrating Biochemistry with Other Subjects

Finally, try to integrate biochemistry with your other studies in dental school, such as physiology and pathology. Recognizing how biochemistry underpins these subjects can create a more cohesive understanding of how your education fits together. For example, while studying the biochemical basis of metabolic disorders, I would link the relevant biochemical processes to their physiological effects and clinical presentations.

By drawing these connections, I could see how biochemistry was not just a standalone subject but a foundational element that impacted various aspects of dental practice.

Mastering biochemistry in dental school doesn't have to be an insurmountable challenge. By employing visual learning techniques, mnemonic devices, active recall, and collaborative study, you can create a rich and engaging learning experience. The key is to find a blend of methods that resonates with your learning style and integrates seamlessly with your overall dental education.

As you embark on this journey, don't hesitate to adapt these strategies to suit your needs. Biochemistry is not just a subject to pass; it's a vital component of your future career as a dental professional. Embrace the challenge, and you'll find that mastering biochemistry will pay off tremendously in your understanding of oral health and patient care.

Tricks and Techniques to Study Dental Materials

Studying dental materials can be both fascinating and daunting, given the intricate details involved in understanding their properties, applications, and implications for clinical practice. However, with the right techniques and strategies, you can effectively master this essential subject. Here are some practical tricks and techniques tailored specifically for dental students to make your study of dental materials more engaging and productive.

1. Utilize Visual Learning Tools

Visual aids can significantly enhance your understanding of dental materials. Consider creating charts, diagrams, and flashcards that outline the properties and uses of various materials. For example, you might create a comparative chart detailing composite resins, glass ionomers, and ceramics, highlighting their mechanical properties, aesthetic qualities, and typical clinical applications.

In my own studies, I used colorful flashcards to memorize key characteristics of each material. On one side, I would write the name of the material, and on the reverse, I'd include its properties, indications, and contraindications. This method not only made review sessions more interactive but also helped reinforce my memory through active recall.

2. Engage in Hands-On Practice

Whenever possible, engage in hands-on practice with dental materials. Many dental schools have simulation labs where you can work with materials like composite resins or impression materials. I remember one lab session where we had to create a direct composite restoration. As I mixed the materials and applied them to a prepared tooth, I gained invaluable insights into the material's handling characteristics and clinical application.

This practical experience allows you to connect theoretical knowledge with real-world applications. Pay attention to how each material behaves during manipulation, curing, and setting. Take notes on your observations to help reinforce your understanding.

3. Group Study Sessions with Focused Topics

Studying dental materials can be enriched through collaborative learning. Forming a study group specifically for this subject can be incredibly beneficial. Organize your sessions around focused topics, such as "Properties of Dental Cements" or "Applications of Impression Materials." Each group member can take responsibility for researching and presenting a specific aspect, fostering a comprehensive discussion.

I recall a particularly effective study session on dental cements where one classmate prepared a presentation on resin cements, while another focused on glass ionomer cements. We shared our findings, discussed clinical scenarios where each type would be appropriate, and even role-played patient interactions to explain our choices. This collaborative approach not only reinforced our learning but also created a more enjoyable atmosphere.

4. Incorporate Case Studies

Case studies provide context and relevance to the study of dental materials. Reviewing real-life clinical scenarios can help you understand how material choices impact patient outcomes. Seek out case studies in your textbooks, academic journals, or online resources.

For example, after learning about the properties of different restorative materials, I came across a case study discussing a patient with extensive caries requiring multiple restorations. The study detailed the decision-making process regarding the choice of materials based on factors like occlusion, aesthetics, and patient preferences. Analyzing these case studies helped me understand the practical implications of material properties in clinical decision-making.

5. Use Mnemonics and Memory Techniques

Given the vast amount of information to retain, memory techniques can be particularly helpful. Create mnemonics to help remember the properties and uses of various dental materials. For example, to remember the key properties of glass ionomer cements—like fluoride release, biocompatibility, and adhesive properties—you could create a phrase like "Fluorescent Bubbles Admire."

Additionally, consider using visual memory techniques, such as the method of loci, where you associate each material with a specific location in a familiar environment, like your home. As you mentally walk through that space, you recall the information associated with each spot.

6. Regular Review and Self-Assessment

Consistency is key when studying dental materials. Schedule regular review sessions to revisit what you've learned. This spaced repetition helps reinforce your memory and understanding. Use self-assessment quizzes or online resources to test your knowledge.

I found it helpful to create practice questions based on the material I studied. For example, after reviewing the characteristics of impression materials, I would quiz myself on their properties, applications, and limitations. This active engagement with the material reinforced my learning and highlighted areas that needed further review.

7. Stay Updated with Current Research

The field of dental materials is continuously evolving, with new products and innovations emerging regularly. Staying updated on current research can provide you with insights into the latest advancements and trends. Subscribe to dental journals or follow relevant online platforms that discuss new materials and technologies.

For instance, I frequently read articles in journals like the Journal of Dental Research or Dental Materials. These readings not only kept me informed but also provided context for my studies, as I could relate what I learned to cutting-edge practices and innovations in dentistry.

Studying dental materials requires a multifaceted approach that combines theoretical knowledge with practical application. By utilizing visual aids, engaging in hands-on practice, collaborating with peers, analyzing case studies, employing memory techniques, and staying current with research, you can enhance your understanding and retention of this crucial subject.

Embrace these strategies, and remember that your journey in mastering dental materials is an essential foundation for your future clinical practice. As you develop your expertise, you will find that your knowledge of materials will not only impact your technical skills but also your ability to make informed decisions that contribute to better patient care. Happy studying!

Tricks and Techniques for Studying Dental Anatomy and Histology

Dental anatomy and histology are foundational subjects in dental education, essential for understanding the structure and function of teeth and their surrounding tissues. Mastering these topics can be challenging due to the intricate details and vast amount of information involved. However, with the right strategies and techniques, you can enhance your learning experience and retention. Here are some effective tricks to study dental anatomy and histology tailored for dental students.

1. Utilize Visual Aids

Both dental anatomy and histology are highly visual subjects. Making use of visual aids can greatly enhance your understanding and retention of the material. Diagrams, models, and histological slides can provide clear representations of complex structures.

For example, I found that using 3D dental models was invaluable when studying the anatomy of teeth. Holding a model in my hands while referring to my textbooks helped me visualize the relationship between different anatomical features, such as cusps, ridges, and the pulp chamber. I also created flashcards with labeled diagrams of teeth, which I could use for quick reviews. On one occasion, I joined a study group where we brought our models and took turns explaining different features. This collaborative effort helped reinforce our learning and made the anatomy come alive.

2. Create Detailed Notes and Summaries

Summarizing your lecture notes and creating detailed study guides can help distill complex information into manageable chunks. As I progressed through my dental anatomy courses, I developed a habit of synthesizing my notes into concise summaries. For instance, after each lecture, I would take time to summarize key concepts, such as the morphology of specific teeth or the development stages of oral tissues.

To make my notes even more effective, I incorporated color coding and diagrams. For example, I would use different colors to highlight enamel, dentin, and pulp in my summaries, making it easier to visually differentiate between these structures. I also included quick reference charts that summarized the main characteristics of each tooth type, which proved useful for exam preparation.

3. Engage in Active Learning Techniques

Active learning techniques, such as teaching others or applying knowledge in practice, can significantly enhance retention. Teaching concepts to a peer or even to yourself out loud forces you to articulate your understanding and identify gaps in your knowledge.

I often formed study pairs with classmates, where we would quiz each other on key topics. For example, while studying histology, we would take turns describing the characteristics of different tissues, like enamel and cementum, and quiz each other on their histological features. This peer-teaching approach not only reinforced my learning but also built confidence in my understanding of the material.

Additionally, applying knowledge in a practical context—such as during lab sessions or clinical simulations—helps solidify your grasp of both anatomy and histology. I remember working in the histology lab, where we examined prepared slides of oral tissues under the microscope. Identifying different types of cells and structures in real slides connected theoretical knowledge with practical application, deepening my understanding.

4. Use Mnemonics and Memory Techniques

Given the vast amount of information in dental anatomy and histology, memory techniques can be lifesavers. Creating mnemonics helps encode complex information into memorable phrases. For example, to remember the order of eruption for primary teeth, I created a phrase: "My First Teeth Come In Many Places" (M for Mandibular, F for First, T for Teeth, C for Canines, I for Incisors, M for Molars, and P for Premolars). This simple phrase helped me recall the eruption order effortlessly.

I also utilized visual mnemonics by associating specific tooth features with memorable images. For example, I imagined molars as "molar mountains" to remember their broad, flat surfaces, while canines were "canine fangs," emphasizing their sharp points. These vivid images made it easier to recall anatomical features during exams.

5. Incorporate Technology and Online Resources

Leverage technology to access a wealth of online resources that can supplement your studies. Educational platforms, YouTube channels, and interactive apps can provide alternative explanations and visualizations that may resonate with your learning style.

During my studies, I frequently used online platforms like SketchyMedical and Osmosis, which offer engaging videos that break down complex topics into digestible content. For histology, I found interactive apps that allowed me to virtually explore histological slides, zooming in on cellular structures to understand their relationships. These resources made learning more dynamic and less daunting.

6. Schedule Regular Review Sessions

Regular review sessions are crucial for long-term retention, especially for subjects that require memorization of numerous details. I found it helpful to create a review schedule that allowed me to revisit topics multiple times before exams.

For instance, I would allocate time each week to revisit different aspects of dental anatomy. One week, I might focus solely on the maxillary teeth, while the next week would be dedicated to mandibular teeth. During these sessions, I would use my summaries and flashcards to reinforce my understanding, ensuring that I was not cramming but instead building a solid foundation of knowledge over time.

Studying dental anatomy and histology can be challenging, but with the right techniques, you can enhance your learning experience and mastery of these subjects. By utilizing visual aids, creating detailed notes, engaging in active learning, employing memory techniques, incorporating technology, and scheduling regular reviews, you can make the study process more effective and enjoyable.

As you embark on this journey, remember that mastering these subjects is not just about memorizing details; it's about understanding the intricate relationships between structure and function in the human body. Embrace the challenges, and don't hesitate to lean on your peers and resources along the way. With dedication and the right strategies, you will thrive in your studies and lay a strong foundation for your future career in dentistry.

Chapter 4: Mastering Exam Preparation in Dental School

Examinations in dental school are uniquely challenging, encompassing written exams, OSCEs (Objective Structured Clinical Examinations), and practical assessments. From efficient study techniques to managing performance anxiety and navigating licensing exams, the journey to success in these high-stakes assessments requires a blend of smart planning, consistent effort, and emotional resilience. In this chapter, we'll explore effective study strategies tailored for dental exams, share tips for both written and practical tests, and reflect on memorable exam moments that taught valuable lessons.

Efficient Study Strategies for Written Exams, OSCEs, and Practical Assessments

Navigating the varied exam formats in dental school can be overwhelming. Each type of exam—whether a written test, OSCE, or practical assessment—demands a tailored approach.

For written exams, the sheer amount of material can be daunting. To manage this, I found that breaking down the syllabus into manageable chunks early on made a difference. I relied heavily on active recall and spaced repetition—two methods that changed my study game. Flashcards became my best friends; instead of just re-reading notes, I quizzed myself on key topics and gradually built up to more complex concepts. Testing myself over time helped move information from short-term memory to long-term understanding.

OSCEs require an entirely different approach, blending theoretical understanding with practical skills. To prepare, I organized sessions with classmates where we would role-play as both clinician and patient, challenging each other with hypothetical questions and unexpected scenarios. Once, a friend posed a question about a rare condition I wasn't well-versed in. I didn't know the answer right away, but I practiced keeping calm, assessing the situation, and logically deducing my approach. These kinds of experiences were invaluable because they taught me to think on my feet, a skill that's vital in real clinical practice.

For practical exams, hands-on practice was essential. I dedicated hours to refining specific skills, such as cavity preparations and impressions. As I practiced, I found that visualize-ation helped me build confidence; mentally running through the steps before I even touched the tools prepared me to execute the task with precision. During one exam, I caught myself feeling rushed, but I stopped, took a breath, and refocused. This moment reinforced the importance of prioritizing quality over speed—a lesson that continues to serve me in my clinical work.

Exam Day Routines, Tips for Performance Anxiety, and Handling Unexpected Questions

The way you approach exam day can have a significant impact on your performance. Developing a routine to minimize stress and keep yourself grounded is essential.

On exam days, my routine started with an early morning walk to center my thoughts, followed by a balanced breakfast to fuel me for the day. Last-minute cramming only increased my stress, so instead, I'd review only flashcards and focus on taking deep breaths to calm any nerves. Visualization was also a powerful tool—I'd imagine myself calmly entering the exam room, fully focused and confident. This visualization exercise became a ritual that set a positive, calm tone.

Managing performance anxiety was a journey. Deep breathing exercises helped me before every OSCE or practical, giving me a moment to ground myself. Another helpful technique was reframing my thoughts. Rather than viewing the examiners as judges, I imagined them as mentors observing my learning. This simple mindset shift transformed the exam environment from intimidating to supportive, allowing me to perform with greater ease.

Dealing with unexpected questions was always a test of composure. During one OSCE, I encountered a question on a rare genetic disorder. Initially, I panicked, but I reminded myself to take a deep breath and think it through. Drawing on general principles, I logically reasoned my response, and while it wasn't perfect, it demonstrated my critical thinking. This experience taught me that it's okay not to know everything; sometimes, showcasing your reasoning process can make a strong impression.

Recollections of High-Stakes Exams and Learning from Mistakes

High-stakes exams in dental school often bring intense pressure, but they also provide some of the most valuable learning experiences. One particularly memorable exam was a practical on restorative dentistry. Despite hours of preparation, exam day nerves got the best of me, and I accidentally fractured the restoration while working on a patient simulation. Initially, I was devastated, but I learned a powerful lesson that day: mistakes are part of learning. What matters most is how you respond. I explained the situation to the examiner, calmly addressed the fracture, and completed the repair. This taught me resilience, patience, and the importance of staying composed—skills that have served me well in both exams and clinical practice.

Study Techniques Specific to Dental Exams

Dental exams cover a wide range of material, from microscopic details of oral histology to procedural steps in clinical practice. Over time, I developed study techniques that catered to the unique demands of these exams.

One effective approach was concept mapping for interconnected subjects. For instance, while studying dental anatomy, I created visual maps linking structures, functions, and clinical implications, helping me not only memorize but understand relationships. This method was particularly useful in practical exams, where questions often require the application of knowledge in real-world scenarios.

For written exams, I used the "Feynman Technique" to explain concepts as though I were teaching them to someone without a medical background. Simplifying complex ideas improved my retention and allowed me to quickly recall information during exams.

In OSCEs and lab exams, repeated practice built muscle memory for each clinical procedure. I focused on memorizing each step, which freed up mental bandwidth to tackle unexpected questions with confidence.

Tips for OSCEs and Lab Exams

In OSCEs and lab exams, where practical skills are evaluated, preparation requires a slightly different approach. Becoming familiar with the checklist for each station, if possible, can clarify what's expected and ease some of the uncertainty.

One memorable OSCE moment taught me the value of adaptability. At a station where I was to demonstrate an injection technique, the tools weren't arranged as I expected. I took a moment to gather myself, mentally adjusted, and proceeded carefully. This experience underscored the importance of flexibility and composure—qualities that are just as crucial as technical skills in clinical practice.

Exam Tips and Tricks

Dental exams come with unique challenges, and these specific strategies proved invaluable in my preparation:

1. Mock Exams with Peers: Simulating exam conditions with classmates created a realistic environment that enhanced my preparation. We took turns acting as examiners, asking each other unexpected questions to push our critical thinking.

2. Using Past Papers: For written exams, practicing with past papers revealed common themes and frequently tested concepts, allowing me to streamline my study focus.

3. Recording Practice Procedures: I recorded myself performing procedures and reviewed the videos to identify areas for improvement. This was especially helpful for exams that demanded clinical precision, allowing me to refine my technique before the real assessment.

Handling Licensing Exams: The Final Hurdle

Licensing exams bring everything full circle, testing the comprehensive knowledge and skills needed for professional practice. Preparing for these exams is demanding but rewarding, requiring a balance of review and practical application.

To stay organized, I created a detailed study schedule that allocated specific time for each major subject, alternating between theoretical review in the mornings and hands-on practice in the afternoons. This schedule kept me focused and ensured I reviewed all essential topics without feeling overwhelmed.

Injecting humor into study sessions helped too. My study group and I would share mnemonics or jokes to lighten the atmosphere. During one session, we even made a parody song about cranial nerves, which left us laughing but also helped solidify the material in a fun way.

Embracing the Journey

Preparing for exams in dental school is more than a test of knowledge; it's a journey of resilience, growth, and transformation. With every exam, you're not only developing clinical skills but also building the qualities needed to become a compassionate and capable dental professional. Embrace the process, learn from each challenge, and remember that every step is bringing you closer to your ultimate goal.

Chapter 5: Understanding Your Clinical Schedule and Requirements

Setting a Strong Foundation for Success

Preparing for clinical postings can be a daunting prospect, but laying out a clear roadmap is one of the best ways to make sure you're set up for success. Knowing what's expected in each clinical rotation helps you not only plan your time effectively but also focus on developing specific skills needed in different dental specialties. Here's how you can take a structured, proactive approach to understanding your clinical schedule and requirements.

Preparing for clinical postings and managing patients effectively are pivotal skills for any dental student. Clinical experience bridges the gap between theory and practice, helping you develop confidence, empathy, and professional competence. Here's a comprehensive guide on how to get the most out of your clinical postings and be ready to handle patient cases smoothly.

1. Thoroughly Review the Syllabus and Clinical Requirements

Before your clinical rotations begin, take time to go over the syllabus and any department-specific requirements. Each rotation will have unique learning goals, so understanding these in advance helps you focus on building the right skills. For example, a posting in periodontics will likely involve scaling, root planing, and assessment of gingival health, whereas a rotation in endodontics will emphasize root canal treatments, pulpal health, and emergency pain management.

Don't just skim through this information—treat it like a roadmap. Look for specific competencies you'll be assessed on. This can include practical skills (like hand instrumentation for scaling), diagnostic abilities (such as identifying different stages of periodontal disease), and even communication skills, such as explaining oral hygiene instructions to patients.

Example Strategy: Say you have a rotation coming up in periodontics. Review the core objectives, including assessment techniques for gum health, recognizing signs of periodontal issues, and practicing procedures like scaling and root planing. Make a checklist of each objective and skill. With this, you can monitor your progress as you move through the rotation, ensuring you're covering all bases.

2. Identify and Prepare for Key Cases You'll Encounter

Once you understand your objectives, the next step is to make a list of the cases you're expected to complete. Clinical postings often come with requirements, such as performing a set number of extractions, restorations, or scaling procedures. Knowing these requirements beforehand allows you to set realistic goals and track your progress over the course of your posting.

Break down this list into specific tasks so that you can gradually work through them. This can help you avoid last-minute stress when nearing the end of your rotation and gives you a clear sense of purpose each day.

Example: If you know you'll need to complete at least five restorative procedures during a restorative dentistry rotation, you could plan to schedule one or two restorations each week. This gives you enough time to focus on quality over quantity while ensuring you meet the required numbers by the end of the posting.

3. Seek Out Resources for Extra Practice in Weak Areas

Clinical rotations are an excellent time to focus on refining skills that you might not feel confident in. Reviewing the rotation's competencies beforehand allows you to pinpoint areas where you might need additional practice. For instance, if you find periodontics challenging, start brushing up on assessment techniques and review anatomy relevant to periodontal treatments.

Consider reaching out to instructors or senior students if you feel uncertain about any specific procedure. This proactive approach shows a willingness to learn and can often lead to valuable advice or additional practice opportunities.

Example: If scaling and root planing are part of your periodontal rotation, and you're not confident with your instrumentation techniques, ask a senior student for tips on hand positioning, or watch tutorial videos on effective instrumentation. Getting comfortable with these skills before you encounter real cases can make you feel more prepared and confident.

4. Set Practical Goals and Track Your Progress

Breaking down your clinical requirements into achievable daily or weekly goals is an effective way to stay on track. Having these smaller targets ensures you're making steady progress without overwhelming yourself, and it allows you to see tangible achievements as you go.

Example: Suppose you have a rotation that requires you to complete a set number of scaling procedures. You might set a goal to complete at least one scaling every two days. If your goal is too ambitious, adjust it—but try to maintain a rhythm that keeps you progressing steadily.

Consider creating a "progress tracker" in a notebook or on your phone where you can jot down what you've achieved each day. This can include the types of cases handled, feedback received, or techniques practiced. Over time, this log not only helps with accountability but also serves as a personal record of growth and skill development.

5. Familiarize Yourself with Rotation-Specific Protocols

Every department will have its own set of protocols—these can range from safety and sanitation protocols to patient management techniques. Knowing these protocols in advance ensures that you're fully prepared and professional from day one.

For example, in a periodontics rotation, sterilization procedures are particularly stringent due to the risk of infection in soft tissues. Familiarize yourself with the protocol for instrument sterilization and the appropriate PPE (personal protective equipment) requirements. This knowledge not only protects you and your patients but also contributes to a smooth, efficient workflow.

If your rotation involves a procedure with multiple steps—such as scaling with ultrasonic instruments—know the exact cleaning and sterilization process to follow afterward. This attention to detail demonstrates professionalism and adherence to high standards of patient care.

Getting prepared for clinical postings takes more than just knowing the theory; it's about organizing yourself, setting clear goals, and continuously building your skills. By thoroughly understanding your clinical schedule and requirements, you're setting a solid foundation for a productive rotation where you'll feel more confident in applying your knowledge practically.

When you enter a rotation well-prepared, you can focus more on refining your skills rather than scrambling to meet requirements. Each day becomes an opportunity for growth as you work toward becoming a capable, compassionate dental professional. Whether it's mastering the art of a perfect scaling technique or understanding how to explain post-procedure care to a patient, the efforts you put into preparing for your clinical rotations will shape you into a well-rounded dentist ready to tackle any challenge.

Brush Up on Theory and Practical Knowledge: Strengthening Your Foundation for Clinical Success

In clinical postings, where real-life patient care takes center stage, the shift from theory to practice can be challenging yet highly rewarding. Clinical environments demand not only a solid foundation in theoretical knowledge but also the ability to adapt that knowledge to real-world situations. A solid grasp of essential subjects like oral pathology, pharmacology, and dental anatomy is key to feeling confident and competent in treating patients. Here's a comprehensive guide to effectively brushing up on your theoretical and practical knowledge to prepare for your rotations.

1. Revisit Core Subjects and Principles

Every clinical rotation has a unique focus, and each requires a specific set of foundational knowledge to perform effectively. Before your posting, invest time in reviewing the basics of the specialty you'll be working in. Going through high-yield topics such as oral pathology, pharmacology, and dental anatomy can provide a refresher and make you feel better equipped to handle what lies ahead.

For instance, if your upcoming rotation is in oral surgery, focusing on the principles of exodontia (tooth extractions), understanding the indications for extractions, and reviewing the complications that may arise during surgical procedures will give you a head start. Spend time on identifying types of impacted teeth, contraindications for extractions, and the use of surgical instruments.

Example Strategy: Say your rotation involves endodontics. Reviewing tooth anatomy, particularly root canal morphology, will prove invaluable when performing procedures like pulp testing or root canal therapy. Go over how different instruments are used in each step of a root canal treatment to solidify your understanding of the process.

2. Review Specialty-Specific Conditions and Treatments

Once you've covered the foundational subjects, delve deeper into conditions and treatments that are most relevant to your specific rotation. Each specialty has its own set of procedures and clinical skills. Reviewing these not only boosts your theoretical knowledge but also helps you mentally prepare for the types of cases you'll see.

Example: If you're starting a periodontics rotation, focus on gum diseases such as gingivitis and periodontitis. Brush up on how to diagnose these conditions by understanding the visual signs and symptoms. Review treatment protocols, such as scaling, root planing, and the use of local antimicrobial agents. Knowing these specifics makes it easier to engage in discussions with your supervisors and feel confident in applying these skills on patients.

Technique for Studying: Use case-based learning to make this process engaging. Instead of just reading about gingivitis and periodontitis, study patient cases that outline symptoms, diagnostic criteria, and treatment options. Imagine you're handling the case yourself and consider what questions you'd ask the patient or what techniques you'd use.

3. Create Quick Reference Tools

Clinical settings can be fast-paced, so having quick reference materials on hand can be incredibly helpful. Preparing resources like flashcards, summary sheets, or checklists for essential procedures or drug dosages will make it easier to look up information on the go. These tools help reinforce memory and serve as valuable aids when you need a quick refresher.

Example: For oral surgery, create flashcards with local anesthesia techniques, commonly used drugs, their dosages, indications, and contraindications. These flashcards will come in handy on rotation, especially if you're new to administering anesthesia independently. You can review them before procedures or even during breaks to reinforce this crucial information.

Tip for Efficiency: Consider using digital flashcard apps such as Anki or Quizlet, which allow you to organize and categorize information for different rotations. You can even create decks specific to each specialty, making it easy to review pertinent information quickly.

4. Practice Procedure Steps Mentally

Visualizing procedures step-by-step can be incredibly helpful in building your confidence and reinforcing the mechanics of different techniques. Before each clinical day, mentally rehearse the steps involved in common procedures. This technique helps bridge the gap between theory and practice, providing a mental roadmap to guide you through real-life applications.

Example: If you're heading into a restorative dentistry rotation, spend time visualizing the process of a cavity preparation or a composite filling. Mentally walk yourself through the steps, from patient positioning and anesthesia to cavity preparation, etching, bonding, and placing the composite. Imagine using each instrument and think about the sensations and sounds involved to help familiarize yourself with the process.

5. Use Visual Aids to Reinforce Anatomy and Techniques

Visual aids can be powerful tools in consolidating anatomical and procedural knowledge. Reviewing diagrams, models, and videos gives you a clearer understanding of spatial relationships within the mouth, which is crucial for procedures involving precision, such as extractions or restorations.

Example: If your rotation is in endodontics, refer to cross-sectional images or models of tooth anatomy, highlighting the different canals and accessory canals. Videos of root canal procedures can also show you the correct angulations, how to negotiate canals, and the application of obturation techniques. Watching these visuals before starting your rotation helps ensure you're not encountering the procedure "blind."

Technique for Visual Learning: Try sketching out anatomical diagrams or procedural steps on paper. Drawing out the anatomy of a molar tooth, for example, can enhance your memory and help you visualize canal positions when performing root canal therapy. Additionally, review surgical videos that emphasize proper instrument handling and procedural flow to prepare you for more hands-on aspects.

6. Conduct Pre-Shift Reviews for Each Posting Day

Making time for a quick, targeted review before each day's clinical posting helps reinforce the material and keeps you prepared for the day's cases. Rather than extensive study sessions, focus on the essentials—such as procedural steps, dosages, or patient handling techniques. This review session can be as short as 10–15 minutes and will help you feel organized and confident.

Example: If you're entering an oral surgery rotation and expect to assist with extractions, review the basic steps of the procedure, from anesthesia to instrument selection and post-extraction instructions. Look up key aspects like incision techniques, bone removal, or suture placement to prepare yourself for possible tasks you may be asked to assist with.

Putting It All Together: Building Confidence Through Preparation

Brushing up on theory and practical knowledge doesn't just prepare you for clinical scenarios—it builds a foundation of confidence and adaptability. Each step of preparation, from reviewing core subjects to creating quick-reference tools, sharpens your skills and equips you for the dynamic environment of clinical rotations.

The time and effort you put into preparing for clinical postings will ultimately translate to more effective patient care and a more enriching learning experience. Not only will you feel more capable of handling clinical tasks, but you'll also find yourself becoming a more independent, skilled dental professional. Embrace the process of learning, revisit foundational concepts often, and remember that each rotation is a stepping stone toward the competence and confidence required to excel in patient care.

Prepare a Clinical Kit and Organize Your Tools: Ensuring Efficiency and Professionalism in Every Patient Interaction

As you enter the clinical phase of dental school, having an organized and well-prepared clinical kit is essential. Being equipped with the right tools not only boosts your confidence but also reflects your professionalism and readiness in front of patients and mentors. This guide offers a comprehensive approach to creating and organizing a clinical kit that will save you time, reduce stress, and enhance your efficiency during each clinical posting.

1. Stock Up on Essential Instruments and Supplies

Each clinical department requires specific instruments and materials, so stocking up on essentials before your posting begins is crucial. For general clinical work, your kit should always include fundamental tools such as mirrors, explorers, probes, and cotton forceps. These are the "bread and butter" of any dental toolkit, and having them readily available helps you avoid delays and lets you focus on patient care.

Core Instruments to Include:

Mirrors: For enhanced visibility and to help retract soft tissues during exams.

Explorers and Probes: Vital for assessing caries, plaque deposits, and periodontal health.

Cotton Forceps: Useful for handling gauze and cotton rolls without breaking sterility.

Additionally, depending on the rotation, your essentials might include items such as anesthesia syringes, burs for cavity preparation, and disposable materials like cotton rolls and gauze. Ensure these items are always stocked in your kit, as running low in the middle of a procedure can disrupt your workflow and patient experience.

Example for Specialty-Specific Preparations:

If you're starting a restorative dentistry rotation, make sure your kit includes filling materials like composite and amalgam, along with the necessary instruments like spatulas, burnishers, and shade guides. Each tool should have its designated place in your kit to streamline the filling procedure, reducing stress and minimizing the chance of errors.

2. Create a "Grab-and-Go" Clinical Bag

The concept of a "grab-and-go" clinical bag is to keep all essential tools and supplies organized and easily accessible, so you're always ready for any patient scenario. This bag is especially useful for unexpected cases or when you're assigned to multiple departments in one day.

Consider segmenting your clinical bag by department, so each set of tools is organized by the procedure type. You can use small, clear pouches for each specialty—endodontics, periodontics, restorative, etc.—and label them accordingly. This way, you won't have to dig through an unorganized bag in search of a specific instrument, saving you valuable time and reducing stress during patient care.

Key Components for a Grab-and-Go Bag:

Basic Kit: Mirror, explorer, cotton forceps, probes, tweezers.

Specialty Kits: For example, a periodontal pouch could include scalers, curettes, and antimicrobial gels; an endodontic pouch might have files, sealers, and irrigation solutions.

Emergency Essentials: Always include a backup mirror, cotton forceps, and an explorer, in case one set becomes contaminated or is misplaced.

Example: On a busy day with rotations in both periodontics and oral surgery, having pre-organized pouches for each specialty makes transitions seamless. You'll only need to switch out the specialty pouches, knowing your tools are already arranged for optimal access.

3. Sterilize and Maintain a Routine for Your Tools

In a clinical setting, sterilization is non-negotiable. Ensuring your tools are sterilized and stored properly not only meets infection control standards but also demonstrates your professionalism. Each morning, check that your instruments are ready to go, neatly organized, and free of contaminants. Maintaining a sterilization log or checklist can be a good habit to develop, especially if you are responsible for multiple sets of instruments in a busy clinic.

Routine Sterilization Protocol:

After Every Patient: Immediately clean and sterilize any tools used, returning them to their designated places in your kit once sterilized.

Daily Checks: Ensure all tools in your clinical bag are sterilized before starting your day. A quick check each morning will prevent any last-minute rushing or tool shortages.

Label and Organize: Use labelled trays or pouches for your instruments. Clear labelling helps both you and the clinic staff quickly identify and access your tools when needed.

Example: After a day of back-to-back restorations, develop the habit of cleaning, sterilizing, and organizing your instruments at the end of the day. Keeping tools in a sterilization pouch overnight ensures they're ready for the next day. This habit can also save you precious minutes in the morning and ensures that each patient starts with sterile, well-maintained instruments.

4. Maintain an Inventory Checklist

Keeping an inventory checklist of your instruments and materials can prevent shortages and help you track what needs replenishment. Running out of an essential item, such as cotton rolls or anesthesia cartridges, in the middle of a procedure can be stressful and inconvenient, so regular inventory checks will keep you well-prepared.

Inventory Essentials:

Disposable Items: Cotton rolls, gauze, rubber dam materials, and suction tips.

Anesthetics and Syringes: Track the expiration dates of anesthetic solutions and replenish as necessary.

Restorative Materials: Make sure composite materials, bonding agents, and other consumables are topped up regularly.

Technique: At the beginning of each week, review your checklist and stock up on any items you're low on. This proactive approach ensures that you have everything you need, even on busier clinic days when restocking might not be feasible.

Example: Suppose you're on an oral surgery rotation that requires regular use of local anesthesia. By keeping a checklist of syringes and anesthetic doses, you'll be aware of how much you have left and can restock without any last-minute stress. Knowing your kit is fully stocked enables you to focus on the patient instead of logistics.

5. Arrange Your Kit in the Order of Use

Organizing your tools in the order of use—often referred to as a "workflow layout"—can make a significant difference in the smoothness and efficiency of your procedures. Arrange your instruments in sequence, with each tool in its specific spot, so you can reach for them in a predictable order. This organized setup reduces the time spent searching for instruments and creates a seamless flow, keeping both you and the patient at ease.

Workflow Layout Example for Restorative Dentistry:

  - Place the mirror, explorer, and cotton forceps/ tweezers at the front for initial examination.

  - Arrange the syringe and anesthesia-related tools next for quick administration.

  - Line up filling materials and instruments like spatulas, carvers, and burnishers in the sequence of their use during a restoration procedure.

  - Lastly, have gauze, cotton rolls, and other finishing materials at the back for easy access.

Practical Example: On the day of a complex restorative procedure, having tools laid out in the order of use can significantly reduce stress. Each instrument should be exactly where you expect it to be, allowing you to work smoothly and focus fully on the patient rather than searching for equipment.

Efficiency and Professionalism Through Preparation

Having a well-organized, ready-to-go clinical kit empowers you to focus on patient care, not logistics. By stocking up on essential instruments, maintaining sterilization routines, creating a grab-and-go bag, and setting up your kit in a workflow-friendly manner, you're setting yourself up for success. These small yet powerful habits build your confidence, reduce stress, and convey a sense of professionalism that patients and mentors will notice.

The investment you make in organizing your clinical kit will pay off by improving both your efficiency and the quality of care you provide. Taking these steps not only ensures you're prepared for each patient but also fosters the habit of staying organized, a valuable skill that will benefit you throughout your dental career.

Observe and Learn from Senior Clinicians: Building Skills through Experience and Mentorship

In the world of dental education, wisdom doesn't just come from books—it's often passed down through the practiced hands and words of seasoned clinicians. As you observe these professionals, remember the proverb: "Experience is the best teacher." By attentively learning from senior residents, professors, and experienced practitioners, you can glean invaluable insights that go beyond textbooks—nuanced techniques, patient interactions, and decision-making strategies that truly shape quality care. Here's how to absorb every ounce of knowledge from these interactions, building a foundation that will stay with you throughout your career.

1. Observe Patient Interactions with a Keen Eye

"Actions speak louder than words." Watching how senior clinicians engage with patients offers lessons in both care and communication. Pay close attention to how they build rapport, address patient concerns, and create a comfortable environment. You'll quickly see that a skilled clinician can put a patient at ease before even picking up an instrument.

Communication Style: Notice how they break down complex procedures into language that patients can understand. They often simplify medical jargon without losing meaning, making patients feel informed and respected.

Empathy and Reassurance: Watch for the subtle ways they handle anxious patients—reassuring words, calm explanations, and nonverbal cues that convey empathy.

Professional Boundaries: Observe how they balance friendliness with professionalism, creating a respectful yet approachable environment.

In one of my rotations, I watched a professor approach a nervous patient needing a root canal. Rather than diving into technical terms, he began by asking about the patient's dental history and comfort levels. This small interaction eased the patient's anxiety, turning the explanation into a conversation instead of a lecture. He used relatable analogies to make the information digestible, reminding me that often, the simplest gestures can have the greatest impact.

2. Study Clinical Techniques with Practical Intent

In the words of an old saying, "A picture is worth a thousand words," and a live demonstration is worth even more. Observing an experienced clinician perform a procedure can reveal countless details that can be challenging to grasp through study alone. Every movement, every tool choice is purposeful. By watching closely, you'll pick up on the refined techniques that years of practice have perfected.

Instrument Handling: See how they hold and manoeuvre instruments with ease, minimizing strain and maximizing control.

Hand Positioning: Observe the stability and precision in their hand placement, especially in complex procedures.

Use of Force and Pressure: Pay attention to how much force they apply—particularly in cases like extractions, where over- or underuse can cause complications.

During my oral surgery rotation, I watched a clinician skillfully perform a difficult extraction. He positioned his non-dominant hand to support the patient's jaw while using his dominant hand with precision. This technique stabilized the jaw, ensuring better control and reducing discomfort for the patient. This observation highlighted how hand support and instrument grip can make a tangible difference, knowledge that a book alone could never fully convey.

3. Absorb Patient Management Strategies

Senior clinicians have a seasoned understanding of patient management, a skill that can't be underestimated. Managing patients effectively—especially anxious ones—takes years of practice. "Smooth seas do not make skillful sailors," and observing clinicians manage challenging situations is a crash course in adaptability and calmness under pressure.

Handling Difficult Situations: Observe how they deal with patients who are apprehensive, resistant, or in pain. Many times, they adjust their approach or take a momentary pause to help the patient feel more at ease.

Time Management: See how they maintain the flow of treatments, even when complications arise.

Educating Patients: Note how they explain preventive care or aftercare, empowering patients to take an active role in their health.

During a periodontal rotation, I watched a resident work with an anxious patient scheduled for scaling. Rather than rushing the process, the resident acknowledged the patient's concerns, walked them through a simple breathing exercise, and then proceeded. This patient-centered approach diffused the tension, allowing the procedure to go smoothly. Observing this situation reinforced the importance of adaptability and patience.

4. Take Notes and Reflect on Each Observation

Keeping detailed notes allows you to internalize what you observe. By reflecting on these notes, you give yourself time to process and integrate new techniques. "A short pencil is better than a long memory." Organized, thoughtful notes can be a priceless reference as you begin to perform these procedures yourself.

Organize by Specialty: Divide your notes into specialties—endodontics, oral surgery, periodontics—making it easy to review later.

Highlight Key Takeaways: After each observation, summarize your notes with actionable takeaways, like "use relatable analogies" or "stabilize hands during extractions."

Set Personal Goals: Challenge yourself to apply these techniques in future patient interactions.

After watching a senior dentist respond to a patient's questions about pain management, I noted, "Explain post-op care using familiar analogies—avoid jargon." Reflecting on these small details made me more prepared and confident when the next patient asked similar questions.

5. Build Relationships and Ask Questions

Remember the proverb, "Ask, and you shall receive." Don't hesitate to engage with clinicians after observing a procedure. Most appreciate inquisitive students and are more than willing to share additional insights and advice. Building rapport and seeking mentorship can enrich your learning and deepen your understanding of patient care.

Sample Questions:

- "How did you develop your approach to explaining procedures?"

- "What techniques do you recommend for managing patient anxiety?"

- "Are there specific skills you'd recommend practicing to improve precision?"

After a challenging root canal procedure, I asked the clinician how he selects file sizes and adjusts angles. He shared tips on tactile sensitivity and visual cues—guidance that proved invaluable the next time I performed a similar procedure myself.

Embracing Observation as a Tool for Growth

Observation is much more than watching; it's active learning in the highest form. Every observation holds the potential to refine your skills and increase your confidence as a budding clinician. By taking detailed notes, reflecting on these experiences, and asking questions, you accumulate a treasure trove of knowledge that can shape your future practice.

Embrace every opportunity to observe, ask, and learn. As you transition from student to clinician, these insights will not only guide you but help you become a compassionate and skilled professional—one who understands that in dentistry, as in life, *"It's the little things that make the biggest difference."

Enhance Communication Skills and Patient Management Techniques

As a dentist, your interactions with patients are as vital as your technical skills. Patients often come into the dental chair with a mix of anxiety, curiosity, and sometimes, fear. Mastering effective communication—rooted in empathy, clarity, and reassurance—not only makes them more comfortable but also establishes a foundation of trust that can enhance your rapport and improve the overall quality of care. Here are strategies, examples, and tips to help you cultivate a patient-centered communication style that resonates with every patient.

Approach with Empathy: A Caring Introduction

Your demeanour from the moment you introduce yourself sets the tone for the entire appointment. Approach patients warmly, with a smile and a gentle handshake, and try to remember small details about previous conversations if they're repeat patients—these small gestures convey that you value them as individuals, not just cases. An introduction that's friendly yet professional—"Hi, I'm Dr. [Your Last Name]. How are you feeling today?"—establishes rapport instantly.

Early in my practice, I met a patient who had severe dental anxiety due to a negative childhood experience. Instead of diving right into the procedure, I took five minutes to ask about their concerns and explained the treatment plan in a relaxed, conversational tone. I even shared a bit about how common dental anxiety is and how I prioritize comfort. This brief investment in empathy and shared understanding resulted in a patient who felt calmer, listened to, and ultimately completed their treatment plan with greater ease.

Suggestion: If a patient appears visibly anxious, consider adapting your tone and language. Sometimes, taking an extra minute to assure them that they're not alone in their worries, and that you're there to ensure they're comfortable, can make all the difference.

Use Simple, Accessible Language

Medical terminology can sound intimidating, especially for patients who are unfamiliar with dental procedures. Avoid technical jargon and instead opt for terms that are straightforward. Describe each step in terms that resonate with the patient's experience, so they can fully understand their treatment without feeling overwhelmed.

For instance, instead of saying, "I'll perform a periodontal scaling and root planing procedure," try, "I'm going to give your gums a deep clean to get rid of any buildup that regular brushing might miss. This helps keep your gums healthy and your teeth strong."

Tip: Using analogies that relate to common experiences can help patients understand complex concepts. For example, comparing plaque removal to dusting a house or maintaining a garden can make oral hygiene sound relatable and less clinical.

Active Listening: Validate Concerns and Offer Reassurance

Listening to patients' concerns is one of the simplest yet most powerful ways to build trust. If a patient expresses discomfort or fear, listen without interrupting, and then acknowledge their feelings. By validating their concerns—whether about pain, time, or cost—you show that you respect them and are invested in their well-being.

Example: For a patient who is afraid of injections, instead of immediately dismissing their fear, say something like, "I understand. Many people feel this way about injections. Here's what we can do to make this as comfortable as possible." Then, outline any options that might help, such as numbing gels, distraction techniques, or taking things slowly.

Demonstrate Calm, Confident Body Language

Your body language communicates as much as your words, especially in a setting where patients are often lying back, and any facial expressions or gestures can be magnified. Keep your posture open; avoid crossing your arms, and make eye contact when appropriate. During procedures, remember that patients pick up on any signs of hesitation or stress, so approach every treatment with calm confidence.

Tip: If a procedure becomes challenging or takes longer than expected, maintain your calm, steady demeanour. Smile when reassuring patients and explain what's happening in a composed, encouraging tone. They're much more likely to stay calm if they see that you're composed and in control.

Reassurance through Small Talk and Step-by-Step Explanations

Patients often feel most relaxed when they feel in control or at least aware of what's happening. Explain the procedure in small steps as you go along, rather than bombarding them with all the details beforehand. This way, they feel involved in the process without feeling overwhelmed.

Example: Instead of saying, "I'll be drilling into your tooth for a few minutes," say, "I'll start by making a small adjustment here, and if at any point you're uncomfortable, let me know so I can pause." This type of language emphasizes that you're attentive to their comfort and willing to adapt to their needs.

Small talk before beginning—about something as light as the weather, recent news, or their favorite local spots—can also be helpful, especially for patients who are clearly nervous. It shifts their focus away from the upcoming procedure and can relax them into the interaction.

Practice Patience with Repeat Explanations

Some patients may need to hear an explanation more than once to fully understand their treatment. Rather than seeing this as a burden, take it as an opportunity to strengthen your communication skills. Repeat information patiently and adjust your language if needed to ensure they're comfortable and informed.

Suggestion: For patients who may be visual learners, use drawings or models to illustrate procedures. Many people find it easier to understand when they can see a visual representation, which helps break down complex information.

Small Reassurances Build Big Trust

During procedures, small, simple reassurances go a long way. Phrases like, "You're doing great," "We're almost done," or "If you need a break, let me know" can keep patients calm and show that you're attentive to their comfort. These reassurances don't take much effort but can profoundly impact how the patient feels during their time in the chair.

Example: If a patient is receiving a filling, gently remind them of the progress throughout. Instead of a vague "We're halfway done," try specifics like, "We've just finished cleaning out the cavity; now we're filling it in, which is the easy part." This breakdown helps them visualize the process and anticipate the end without feeling anxious.

Conclude with Positive Reinforcement and Aftercare Guidance

When you finish a procedure, offer words of encouragement to make patients feel they've been active participants in their own health. "You did great!" or "You took excellent care of your teeth—let's keep it that way" boosts their confidence and reinforces the idea that maintaining good oral health is a collaborative effort. Be specific when discussing aftercare, but keep it simple.

Example: If a patient has just undergone a cleaning, reinforce good habits by saying, "Your gums look healthier already! Just keep up the brushing and flossing like we talked about, and they'll stay that way." This positive feedback not only boosts their morale but motivates them to maintain those habits between visits.

Build Long-Term Patient Relationships with Follow-Up and Personal Touches

Following up with patients after significant procedures can show them that you genuinely care. A quick call or text to check on their recovery can be immensely reassuring and build loyalty. If your clinic has the resources, sending automated reminders for routine check-ups or anniversaries of their first appointment can make patients feel valued.

Tip: During appointments, take mental notes of any personal details they share (like a recent trip or their pet's name). Mentioning these in future visits—"How was your vacation to Hawaii?"—adds a personalized touch that patients will remember.

Transforming Technical Skill into Compassionate Care

Becoming a caring, communicative dentist is an art as much as a science. By approaching each interaction with empathy, using accessible language, maintaining open body language, and offering reassuring comments, you can significantly improve your patients' experiences. Over time, these efforts in communication and patient management won't just enhance your technical work; they'll build strong, trusting relationships that make patients feel comfortable and valued under your care. After all, as the saying goes, "People don't care how much you know until they know how much you care."

Developing a Treatment Flow and Staying Calm Under Pressure

In a dental practice, managing multiple patients, complex procedures, and sometimes unpredictable scenarios is the norm. Having a structured treatment flow and techniques to remain calm under pressure are essential not only for delivering quality care but also for building confidence in yourself as a clinician. When you establish a consistent, step-by-step approach to each procedure, you allow your mind and body to stay centered and focused, reducing the risk of errors and enabling you to handle challenges more gracefully. Here's how to develop a reliable treatment flow and adopt strategies to stay composed, even during high-pressure situations.

Build a Systematic Treatment Flow: Turning Chaos into Routine

Dentistry involves many complex, high-stakes tasks that demand absolute precision. Breaking down each procedure into manageable steps allows you to move from one phase to the next with clarity, giving you control over even the most challenging treatments. This systematic approach also reassures patients; when they see you following a smooth, predictable routine, they feel more confident in your expertise and less anxious about the process.

For example, if you're performing a filling, establish a flow that can guide you through every stage, even under pressure. Start with anesthesia, checking in with the patient as it takes effect. Then, move to isolation, protecting the surrounding teeth and soft tissues. Follow this by carefully removing decay, keeping your instruments steady and your focus unwavering. Placing the filling becomes another mindful step, ensuring that it's secure and aesthetically pleasing, before moving to the final polish for a smooth, clean result. Each of these steps acts as a checkpoint, creating a rhythm that keeps you grounded.

Tip: Think of each procedure as a dance with specific movements that lead to a predictable, successful outcome. Even when unexpected complications arise, you'll have the muscle memory and confidence to handle them by falling back on your established steps.

Visualization Techniques: Mentally Rehearse the Procedure

One effective way to prepare yourself, especially for complex procedures, is to mentally walk through each step before you even touch an instrument. Visualization helps solidify your treatment flow and gives you a mental rehearsal that calms your nerves, reinforcing both your confidence and your focus.

Example: Suppose you have a challenging extraction ahead. In the minutes before the procedure, close your eyes and picture every step in vivid detail—from positioning the patient and applying anesthesia to selecting the right forceps and visualizing exactly how you'll apply pressure. Imagine the sensation of removing the tooth and the sight of a clean extraction site afterward. This preemptive walk-through reduces the chance of surprises and primes your mind to stay calm and focused.

Many athletes use similar visualization techniques before high-stakes events, picturing every movement and anticipating potential setbacks. As a dentist, visualizing each stage of a procedure helps you respond confidently, as if you've already practiced it in real-time.

Staying Grounded: The Power of Mindfulness and Deep Breathing

It's natural to feel tension, especially when faced with difficult procedures or an anxious patient. Developing simple mindfulness practices can help you reset and maintain your calm, no matter the situation. Practicing deep breathing exercises or grounding techniques before a procedure, or even during a brief pause, can clear your mind, lower your heart rate, and bring your focus back to the task at hand.

Mindfulness Exercise: If you feel the adrenaline rising, take three slow, deep breaths, focusing on your breathing. Inhale for a count of four, hold for four, then exhale slowly for six. This method brings your nervous system back to a calm state, helping you perform with a steady hand and a clear mind. You could also try a grounding technique, like feeling the floor beneath your feet or focusing on the weight of your hands. These small acts pull you out of a stress spiral and anchor you to the present moment.

Prepare for the Unexpected with a "Plan B" Mindset

Even with the best preparation, dentistry often surprises us. A filling may turn out deeper than expected, or a tooth extraction might present additional challenges. Anticipating these potential issues and having a flexible, adaptable mindset will help you pivot gracefully when things don't go as planned.

When preparing for a procedure, quickly review your "Plan B" options, such as alternative techniques, backup tools, or extra anesthesia if needed. Having these backup plans in mind reduces hesitation and enhances your problem-solving skills. You'll also come across as more confident to the patient, which is vital for maintaining their trust.

Example: In a difficult root canal, you may encounter unexpected bleeding or a narrow canal that's tough to access. If you've mentally prepared for such possibilities, you can move seamlessly into alternative strategies without breaking concentration. The patient will likely remain calm as well, seeing your steady, capable approach.

Use Reassuring Body Language to Project Calm

As a dentist, your body language speaks volumes. Even if you feel tense inside, maintaining a relaxed, composed exterior can comfort your patient and keep you grounded. Notice your facial expressions, posture, and movements. Move slowly and deliberately, and keep your shoulders relaxed.

Patients are perceptive, and they can sense your stress, which may amplify their own. A calm, steady demeanor—even if you're mentally working through challenges—reassures patients and allows you to maintain focus. When you find yourself feeling rushed or pressured, pause, adjust your posture, and let your breathing settle before continuing.

Seek Support from Your Team

Don't underestimate the power of teamwork in creating a calm and organized environment. Relying on your dental assistants and other staff to support your treatment flow can ease the workload, reduce stress, and keep you on track. Clear communication with your team before and during a procedure ensures everyone knows their roles and responsibilities, contributing to a smoother experience.

Tip: Before a complex procedure, conduct a quick briefing with your assistant. Discuss the steps you'll take and any anticipated challenges, so your team knows what to expect and can step in with exactly what you need when you need it.

Post-Procedure Reflection: Building Confidence and Experience

After a procedure, take a moment to reflect on what went well and what could be improved. This reflection allows you to continuously refine your treatment flow and identify areas where you can stay calmer or be more efficient. Over time, this practice builds a strong foundation of experience, so that even the most complex treatments feel manageable.

Early in my practice, I found extractions nerve-wracking. I'd always worry about applying too much or too little pressure, which sometimes caused the procedure to take longer than expected. After each extraction, I'd reflect on the technique and think about where I could have adjusted my approach. With time and consistent reflection, I began to find my rhythm, and now extractions are among the procedures I feel most confident handling. This growth only came from taking the time to learn from each experience.

Mastery in Dentistry through Consistent Flow and Composure

In dentistry, staying calm and composed under pressure transforms difficult tasks into manageable, even routine, experiences. By establishing a structured treatment flow, practicing visualization, and utilizing mindfulness techniques, you can approach each procedure with confidence and clarity. Coupled with patient-centered communication, this calm approach reassures your patients and builds their trust, while your steady hands and systematic process ensure top-quality care. Over time, these habits not only enhance your clinical skill but help you develop into a resilient, confident, and highly effective dentist.

Stay Informed on Infection Control Protocols

Infection control is more than a routine protocol—it's a pillar of safe and ethical dental practice. Every action you take to maintain a sterile, hygienic environment speaks to your commitment to patient safety and well-being. For patients, especially those who are already nervous or vulnerable, seeing a dentist who prioritizes infection control instills confidence and trust. Being informed on the latest standards and rigorously applying them ensures that both you and your patients are protected from risks associated with contamination, making your practice a safe haven for everyone involved.

The Importance of Infection Control in Dentistry

Dentistry involves close contact with patients, which inherently carries a higher risk of transmitting pathogens. Saliva, blood, and other bodily fluids can expose both the patient and the clinician to potentially infectious materials, from bacteria and viruses to blood borne pathogens. Understanding infection control is therefore essential, not only to comply with regulations but to create a culture of safety within the practice. When you consistently follow protocols, you reduce the risk of infections, build trust, and foster an environment of respect.

Infection control covers several key areas: sterilization, personal protective equipment (PPE), hand hygiene, and waste management. Each of these protocols has specific steps that, when rigorously adhered to, create a robust defense against infection.

1. Mastering Sterilization: A Non-Negotiable Standard

Sterilization is the first line of defense in infection control. Every instrument that comes into contact with bodily fluids must be properly sterilized before being used on the next patient. Dental instruments such as handpieces, scalers, and probes need to go through a strict sterilization cycle that includes cleaning, disinfecting, and autoclaving.

The autoclave, which uses high-pressure steam, is a dentist's best friend in this regard. Learning to properly load and operate an autoclave, and monitoring it regularly, ensures that instruments are sterilized at the correct temperature and pressure. Any shortcuts in this process can compromise instrument sterility and put patients at risk. Being thorough with sterilization reflects not only your commitment to safety but also your respect for each individual patient.

Imagine a busy day with back-to-back appointments. It might be tempting to skip a step in the sterilization process or rush through it. However, taking the extra time to ensure every instrument is properly sterilized is essential. Over time, your diligence in this area becomes second nature, creating a standard of care that reassures your patients and aligns with the ethics of healthcare.

2. Personal Protective Equipment (PPE): Your Barrier to Transmission

Using PPE is crucial for creating a barrier against infectious agents. Every time you meet a patient, you're potentially exposed to aerosols, droplets, and other forms of contamination. PPE, including gloves, masks, protective eyewear, gowns, and face shields, protects both you and your patients by minimizing direct contact with these pathogens.

While wearing PPE may feel cumbersome, especially during long procedures, it's important to remember that these barriers are protecting your health and your patients. Additionally, ensuring that your PPE is correctly fitted—such as masks that seal well around your nose and mouth—maximizes its effectiveness. When patients see you taking these precautions, they feel safer and more assured about their health in your hands.

Tip: Get into the habit of changing gloves between every patient and even during procedures if you touch a non-sterile surface. Consistency in these habits prevents cross-contamination and maintains the highest standard of infection control.

3. Hand Hygiene: The Cornerstone of Infection Prevention

Hand hygiene might sound simple, but it's one of the most effective ways to prevent the spread of infection. Regular and thorough handwashing removes transient microorganisms that can easily transfer to patients or instruments. The World Health Organization (WHO) recommends washing hands with soap and water for at least 20 seconds, especially before and after each patient.

In a busy dental setting, maintaining hand hygiene requires diligence. Many practitioners use alcohol-based hand sanitizers in situations where a full wash isn't feasible. Hand hygiene is particularly critical when working with vulnerable populations, such as elderly patients or those with compromised immune systems. By making hand hygiene a visible habit, you also communicate to your patients that you take their health seriously.

One way to ensure hand hygiene remains a priority is to create a ritual around it. For instance, as you prepare for a new patient, washing your hands becomes part of your mental preparation for the procedure. This small act not only cleanses your hands but also signals a transition into focusing on the patient's care.

4. Managing Instruments: Safe Handling and Disposal

Proper handling of contaminated instruments is essential for avoiding accidental exposure and ensuring effective sterilization. Develop a routine for managing instruments as soon as they're used, placing them in a designated container for contaminated items. Avoid direct handling of sharp instruments, and use puncture-proof containers to prevent needle-stick injuries.

In addition, waste management plays a crucial role in infection control. Biohazardous waste, such as used gloves, gauze, and any materials that have come into contact with bodily fluids, should be disposed of in biohazard bags. Regularly reviewing and updating your waste disposal practices ensures compliance with regulations and helps keep your clinic environment safe.

Imagine a scenario where a tool slips or a small piece of gauze falls onto a non-sterile surface during a procedure. Instead of reusing it, dispose of it properly and replace it with a sterile item. This might seem wasteful, but it's crucial for infection control. Patients notice this attention to detail and feel reassured that you're prioritizing their safety.

5. Rubber Dam Usage: A Barrier Against Cross-Contamination

Using a rubber dam during procedures like root canals or endodontic treatments is an effective way to isolate the treatment area and prevent contamination. Rubber dams keep saliva and other fluids away from the tooth you're working on, creating a cleaner environment. They also protect patients from accidentally swallowing or inhaling small particles or tools.

Applying rubber dams requires practice, especially for patients with small mouths or challenging anatomy. But once you're comfortable, they become a valuable tool for both infection control and patient comfort.

Example: When performing a root canal, you might explain to the patient that the rubber dam helps create a "dry and clean area" for you to work on and prevents contamination. This not only keeps them informed but also reassures them that you're following best practices.

The Impact of Following Infection Control Protocols: Building Trust and Professionalism

Infection control protocols go beyond mere compliance—they demonstrate professionalism and respect for the health of each patient. When patients see you consistently following stringent protocols, they perceive you as a diligent, caring professional who values their safety. For many patients, seeing this level of commitment to hygiene can make them feel more comfortable and confident in your care.

One dentist shared how his diligence with infection control changed a patient's entire outlook. The patient had been hesitant about dental visits due to a previous experience with an unsterile practice. Observing this new dentist's careful handwashing, changing of gloves, and meticulous handling of instruments convinced the patient to trust dental care again. It was a reminder that these routines, while sometimes tedious, can profoundly affect how patients view their dental experience.

Staying Updated: Infection Control as a Continuous Learning Process

Infection control practices evolve with advancements in medical research, emerging pathogens, and new regulations. Staying informed on the latest updates helps you maintain the highest standard of care. Attending workshops, reviewing updates from the Centers for Disease Control and Prevention (CDC), and engaging in continuing education are excellent ways to stay current.

Being proactive in infection control is more than a checklist; it's an ethical commitment to your patients and yourself. Regularly revisiting your practices and remaining open to learning ensures that your clinic environment remains a place of safety and healing.

Infection Control as a Reflection of Care

Infection control protocols represent the invisible yet powerful aspect of patient care. Every precaution you take—from wearing fresh gloves to managing biohazardous waste—builds a foundation of trust, demonstrating to your patients that you're committed to their safety and well-being. This attentiveness is integral to your identity as a healthcare provider and a key factor in maintaining professionalism in dental practice. By consistently following these protocols, you not only protect your patients and yourself but also reinforce the values of respect, safety, and empathy in the care you provide.

Ask for Feedback and Reflect on Each Patient Case

Feedback and self-reflection are essential to growing as a dentist. Embracing both as part of your routine enables you to continually refine your skills, become more attuned to your patients, and deepen your understanding of each procedure. Asking for feedback from supervisors and experienced colleagues is invaluable, as it provides insights you might miss on your own. Meanwhile, reflecting on each case helps you pinpoint both successes and areas for improvement, solidifying lessons learned in real clinical contexts.

The Importance of Feedback: A Path to Growth and Mastery

When you're in the early stages of clinical practice, every step, gesture, and decision is part of your learning curve. Seeking feedback, especially from instructors or experienced practitioners, allows you to gain perspective on your technique and approach. Even small adjustments—like a tweak in hand positioning or a change in patient interaction—can significantly impact your efficiency and patient comfort.

Being open to constructive criticism can sometimes feel vulnerable, but embracing it as a tool for growth is transformative. Supervisors often see things we don't notice ourselves, and their insights can lead to breakthroughs. When you ask for feedback, you also demonstrate your commitment to self-improvement, a quality that is reassuring to both mentors and patients alike.

Imagine you've just completed a restoration. You might ask your instructor, "Do you think I could have improved any part of that procedure?" They might suggest positioning yourself at a slightly different angle to gain better visibility, or they could point out that a lighter hand pressure would yield better results. Implementing these tips in your next case enhances your skill, ultimately contributing to more seamless and comfortable experiences for your patients.

Cultivating Reflection: Making Each Case a Learning Experience

Reflection is a quiet but powerful tool for self-assessment. After each case, take a moment to ask yourself a few key questions: What went well? What didn't go as planned? Did the patient seem comfortable, and if not, what could you have done differently? These reflections help you mentally review the case, locking in successes and noting areas for future attention.

When you reflect, you're essentially running a post-procedure "debrief" with yourself, identifying strategies to try next time or habits to break. It's a way to improve incrementally with each patient, making adjustments that contribute to the overall quality of your care.

Suppose you're assisting with a patient who seemed anxious during the procedure. Afterward, reflect on whether your words or actions helped ease their anxiety or if there were moments when you could have been more comforting. Perhaps next time, you decide to explain the procedure more slowly or ask more questions to check on their comfort levels. This simple self-assessment keeps you connected to each patient's experience and allows you to fine-tune your approach for future cases.

Seeking Specific Feedback: Going Beyond General Observations

General feedback—like "Good job" or "That went well"—is positive but may not give you actionable insights. To improve effectively, seek specific feedback. Ask questions that help your supervisors focus on particular areas of your technique, such as your handling of instruments, patient communication, or procedural efficiency. By asking targeted questions, you can gain clarity on your strengths and receive practical suggestions for improvement.

Tip: Try to ask one or two specific questions after each case, such as "Is there a better way I could have positioned my hand for that step?" or "Was I clear in explaining the procedure to the patient?" Over time, this habit builds a library of practical advice that can profoundly shape your clinical approach.

Learning from Mistakes: Turning Challenges into Opportunities

Mistakes in clinical settings are natural parts of the learning journey. When something doesn't go as planned, rather than focusing solely on the error, try to see it as a learning opportunity. Reflecting on why it happened, how you reacted, and what you can do differently next time fosters a proactive approach to self-improvement.

For example, if you struggled with achieving a smooth restoration finish, review the steps you took and identify where you might have deviated. It could be as simple as needing a more controlled hand pressure or using a different instrument. Analyzing these moments rather than shying away from them strengthens your resilience and helps prevent similar mistakes in the future.

Say you had a challenging experience with a patient who became uncomfortable during an extraction. Instead of solely feeling frustrated, reflect on what contributed to their discomfort. Was it a lack of reassurance? Were they not properly informed of the steps? Next time, you might decide to spend an extra minute explaining the procedure, allowing the patient to feel more in control and at ease.

Patient Comfort and Communication: Small Adjustments, Big Impacts

Patient interaction and communication are just as vital as technical skills. Reflecting on each patient's demeanor and reactions during treatment can reveal valuable insights. For example, if you notice that a patient appeared tense, you might consider ways to make future interactions more reassuring. It could be as simple as asking them periodically if they're comfortable or adjusting your tone to be more calming.

Patients often feel vulnerable during dental procedures, and acknowledging this vulnerability by reflecting on their comfort level can make a huge difference in how they perceive their experience. Small adjustments, like explaining each step before performing it or using a softer tone, help build trust and alleviate patient anxiety.

You may have a patient who seemed unusually quiet and tense. Reflect on whether you gave them enough information before beginning the procedure. Perhaps next time, you'll make an effort to introduce each step verbally, explaining why you're doing it and what sensations they might feel. Over time, these small adjustments add up to create a more reassuring patient experience, which can be particularly helpful in reducing dental anxiety.

Documenting Reflections: Building a Personal Learning Portfolio

Maintaining a record of your reflections can be immensely helpful. By jotting down your observations after each case, you create a personal portfolio of insights and lessons learned. This not only helps you track your progress but also enables you to revisit challenges and improvements over time.

Documenting reflections can be as simple as keeping a small notebook or digital file where you note key takeaways from each case. This habit of documentation allows you to observe patterns, track your growth, and reinforce positive practices, gradually solidifying your expertise and confidence.

Tip: Try to make brief notes after each case, including what went well, areas for improvement, and any feedback you received. Over time, this "learning log" becomes a valuable resource for reflection and growth.

The Value of Constructive Criticism: Building Resilience and Adaptability

Constructive criticism isn't always easy to hear, but it's one of the fastest routes to mastery. Accepting feedback gracefully and using it as a stepping stone to improve builds resilience and adaptability. When supervisors or mentors point out areas for improvement, rather than feeling discouraged, use it as an opportunity to develop and refine your skills.

Every piece of constructive criticism strengthens your adaptability, an essential trait in a field where every patient and procedure presents a unique set of challenges. Learning to respond positively to feedback equips you to handle a variety of cases with confidence.

The Power of Small Improvements: Growth Through Reflection

By seeking feedback and reflecting on each case, you're setting yourself on a path of continuous improvement. The key to becoming a skilled dentist lies in these incremental gains. Over time, the small insights and adjustments you make each day accumulate, transforming you into a clinician who is both competent and compassionate.

Embracing Feedback and Reflection as Tools for Excellence

Being open to feedback and committed to self-reflection are hallmarks of a dedicated healthcare provider. Each patient case provides you with a unique opportunity to learn, whether from successes or challenges. By embracing constructive criticism, reflecting deeply on each experience, and making small, consistent improvements, you develop both your technical skills and your ability to connect with patients. This process of continuous refinement, driven by self-awareness and a willingness to grow, ultimately shapes you into a thoughtful, capable, and caring dentist who inspires trust and comfort in each patient.

Document Your Cases and Create Study Notes

Documenting your clinical experiences and creating study notes are powerful practices that not only enhance your learning but also serve as a roadmap for your growth as a dentist. By meticulously recording your cases, you develop a rich resource that can guide your future practice and help you retain knowledge more effectively.

The Value of Case Documentation: Building a Personal Clinical Library

Every patient interaction is an opportunity to learn. Keeping a log of the cases you handle during your clinical postings allows you to capture the essence of each experience. In this log, note down the procedures performed, the materials used, the patient reactions, and the outcomes. This comprehensive record serves multiple purposes: it helps you identify patterns in your clinical practice, track your progress over time, and reflect on your learning journey.

Consider your case log as a personal clinical library. Each entry is a chapter that chronicles your development, illustrating the diversity of cases you've encountered and the skills you've acquired. Over time, you'll be able to look back and see how far you've come, which can be incredibly motivating and affirming.

Example: After a particularly challenging root canal, take a moment to document your experience. Write down the steps you followed, including any specific techniques you used, the materials you selected, and the rationale behind your choices. Reflect on any difficulties you encountered—perhaps you struggled with achieving proper anesthesia or had to navigate an unusually curved canal. Describe how you managed those challenges. This record not only solidifies your learning but also provides a valuable reference when preparing for exams or approaching similar cases in the future.

Creating Study Notes: Tailoring Your Learning Experience

In addition to your case logs, creating concise study notes on clinical procedures is an excellent way to reinforce your learning. These notes can cover various topics, from extraction techniques to the intricacies of root canal therapy. By distilling complex information into manageable chunks, you make it easier to review and recall when needed.

Personalized study notes are particularly beneficial because they reflect your unique learning experiences. For instance, if you found a specific method particularly effective during an extraction, note it down. If a supervisor provided you with a helpful tip or trick, capture that insight in your notes. Over time, these tailored references can become invaluable resources, showcasing not just textbook knowledge but also the practical wisdom gained through hands-on experience.

Example: After performing an extraction, take a few minutes to jot down the key steps involved. Include specifics about the instruments used, any notable anatomical considerations, and how you managed the patient's comfort throughout the procedure. If a certain technique helped you secure the tooth more efficiently, be sure to highlight that. These notes will serve as quick reminders and refreshers, especially during exam preparations or before a similar procedure.

Patterns and Progress: Analyzing Your Growth

As you build your collection of case logs and study notes, take time to analyze the patterns that emerge. Are there particular types of procedures you find challenging? Do certain patient demographics react differently to treatment? By recognizing these trends, you can tailor your learning and practice to address your areas for improvement.

For instance, if you notice that you struggle more with endodontic procedures, you can dedicate extra study time to mastering those techniques. Conversely, if you excel in patient management, document the strategies that work for you, ensuring you continue to use and refine those approaches.

Collaboration and Sharing Knowledge

In addition to your personal notes, consider sharing your documented cases with peers or mentors. Collaborating in this way can deepen your understanding and open the door to new insights. Discussing your experiences and hearing others' perspectives helps you broaden your knowledge base and enhances your problem-solving skills.

For instance, if a colleague has handled a similar case, their experiences and techniques could provide you with new strategies to consider in the future. Conversely, explaining your approach to a challenging case can reinforce your understanding and help you articulate the rationale behind your choices.

Documenting Challenges and Solutions: Turning Obstacles into Learning Opportunities

Every dentist encounters challenging situations, and how you document these challenges can significantly influence your development. When faced with difficulties during a procedure, make it a habit to note not only what went wrong but also how you resolved the issue. This reflective practice fosters resilience and critical thinking.

Imagine you encounter a complication during a surgical extraction, such as a fractured root. Rather than simply documenting the issue, also write down how you addressed it— perhaps you consulted with a senior colleague for advice or utilized specific instruments to aid in the extraction. This comprehensive documentation serves as a roadmap for similar future challenges, transforming obstacles into valuable learning experiences.

The Role of Reflection: Learning from Each Case

In addition to documenting procedures and outcomes, reflecting on your experiences is key to deepening your learning. After logging a case, take a moment to think critically about what you did well and where you could improve. Did you communicate effectively with the patient? Were there aspects of your technique that felt uncertain? This reflection enables you to internalize your experiences and use them as a foundation for future practice.

Building Confidence Through Documentation

The act of documenting your cases and creating study notes can also build your confidence. As you review your progress and see how you've tackled different challenges over time, you develop a sense of mastery. This growing confidence will enhance your interactions with patients, as you will be better equipped to answer their questions and address their concerns.

Tip: Schedule regular times to review your case logs and study notes. This practice reinforces your learning and allows you to track your growth over time. As you reflect on your journey, you'll be amazed at how far you've come.

A Journey of Continuous Learning and Growth

Documenting your cases and creating study notes are essential practices for any aspiring dentist. By maintaining a detailed record of your clinical experiences, you build a comprehensive resource that supports your ongoing learning journey. These logs and notes not only serve as invaluable references for future cases and examinations but also reflect your growth as a clinician. Through this documentation, you transform each experience into a stepping stone toward greater expertise and confidence, ultimately enhancing your ability to provide exceptional care to your patients. Embrace this journey of continuous learning, and watch as it shapes you into the skilled and compassionate dentist you aspire to be.

Build Your Confidence Gradually

Building confidence as a dental student and clinician is a journey that requires patience, practice, and a willingness to embrace learning opportunities. As you navigate through the complexities of patient care and clinical procedures, it's essential to recognize that confidence is not an inherent trait but a skill that develops over time through experience and reflection.

The Importance of a Gradual Approach: Taking Small Steps

Starting with simpler cases and procedures is a foundational strategy for developing your confidence. This approach allows you to familiarize yourself with clinical environments and the nuances of patient care without feeling overwhelmed. By gradually increasing your level of responsibility, you give yourself the space to learn and grow at a comfortable pace.

Imagine beginning your clinical experience by assisting with routine cleanings and examinations. During these initial encounters, you'll gain valuable exposure to patient interactions, learn to perform basic procedures, and understand how to navigate the dental environment. Each successful cleaning you perform or examination you assist with is a small victory, contributing to your overall sense of competence.

As you master these foundational skills, you can gradually transition to more complex treatments. After becoming comfortable with cleanings, you might move on to helping with basic restorative work, such as applying sealants or doing simple fillings. Each new challenge builds on your existing knowledge and prepares you for the next level of responsibility, like performing extractions or more intricate restorative procedures.

Learning from Mistakes: Embracing Challenges as Growth Opportunities

Mistakes are an inevitable part of the learning process. Accepting this fact early on will help you develop resilience and a growth mindset. Instead of viewing mistakes as failures, reframe them as opportunities to learn and improve. Each error provides valuable feedback that can guide your development and enhance your skills.

When you encounter a challenge or make a mistake, take a moment to reflect on the experience. What went wrong? What could you have done differently? Seeking guidance from mentors or more experienced colleagues is also crucial at this stage. Their insights can provide you with new perspectives and strategies to avoid similar pitfalls in the future.

Let's say you're assisting with a restoration and encounter difficulty in properly isolating the tooth. Instead of becoming discouraged, take a breath and reflect on the situation. Perhaps you realize that you could improve your technique or equipment selection. After the procedure, don't hesitate to ask your supervisor for feedback. They might suggest a different isolation technique or offer tips on how to enhance your approach, transforming a frustrating moment into a valuable learning experience.

Building on Success: Celebrating Small Wins

As you progress through your clinical training, it's essential to celebrate your successes—no matter how small they may seem. Acknowledging your accomplishments, whether it's mastering a technique or receiving positive feedback from a patient, reinforces your growing confidence.

For examples, after successfully performing your first filling, take a moment to reflect on the achievement. Consider how far you've come from your initial days in the clinic when you may have felt unsure about even the simplest procedures. Share this success with your peers or mentors; their encouragement can amplify your sense of accomplishment and motivate you to tackle the next challenge.

The Role of Reflection: Learning from Each Experience

In addition to celebrating your successes, regular reflection is vital for building confidence. After each clinical encounter, take a few moments to think critically about what you did well and what you could improve upon. This reflective practice helps reinforce your learning and solidifies your understanding of various procedures.

For instance, after completing a procedure, you might ask yourself questions like:

- What techniques worked well for me today?

- Did I communicate effectively with the patient?

- Were there any moments of uncertainty, and how can I address them in the future?

By analyzing your experiences, you create a feedback loop that encourages continuous growth and learning.

Setting Realistic Goals: Creating a Roadmap for Progress

To build confidence systematically, consider setting realistic and achievable goals for yourself. Break down your larger aspirations into smaller, manageable steps. For instance, if you aim to master extractions, set incremental goals such as observing experienced dentists, assisting in extractions, and eventually performing them under supervision.

These goals will provide you with a clear roadmap for your progress and allow you to track your development over time. Regularly revisiting your goals helps maintain your motivation and keeps you focused on your growth trajectory.

For example, if your goal is to become proficient in endodontic procedures, you might start by watching videos, then observing procedures, and later assisting. Once you feel confident, you can attempt your first root canal under supervision, applying everything you've learned. Celebrate each achievement, and as you check off your goals, your confidence will naturally grow.

Cultivating a Supportive Environment: Building Your Network

Surrounding yourself with a supportive network is crucial for your confidence-building journey. Engage with your peers, mentors, and instructors who encourage and challenge you to step outside your comfort zone. Sharing experiences and seeking advice from others can bolster your confidence and help you navigate the ups and downs of clinical training.

Consider joining study groups or participating in peer-to-peer discussions where you can share insights and learn from one another's experiences. This collaborative environment fosters a sense of camaraderie and encourages you to grow together.

For instance, participate in group discussions or study sessions where you can practice explaining procedures to your peers. Teaching others reinforces your understanding and boosts your confidence in articulating clinical concepts. You might find that your explanations lead to valuable discussions and new insights, further enhancing your skills.

Confidence as a Journey

Building confidence as a dentist is a gradual process that requires intentionality, reflection, and a willingness to learn from every experience. By starting with simpler cases, embracing mistakes as learning opportunities, celebrating your successes, and setting realistic goals, you can cultivate the confidence needed to thrive in clinical practice.

Remember, every experienced dentist was once in your shoes, navigating the complexities of patient care and mastering their skills. As you move forward on this journey, be patient with yourself, seek guidance, and celebrate your growth. With time, practice, and dedication, you'll transform into a skilled and confident clinician, ready to provide exceptional care to your patients.

In Summary,

Preparation for clinical postings and patient management extends beyond technical skills to encompass communication, organization, and emotional readiness. By balancing study and hands-on practice, developing a systematic approach to each patient, and cultivating empathy and confidence, you'll be well-prepared for your clinical journey in dental school. This experience is a vital step in becoming a competent, compassionate dental professional, equipped to handle the diverse needs of future patients.

Chapter 6: Overcoming Procrastination

Procrastination is a common struggle among dental students, often fueled by the overwhelming workload, high-stakes assessments, and the constant need to balance practical training with theoretical studies. In this chapter, we'll explore how to identify triggers of procrastination, develop effective strategies to combat it, and share personal experiences that highlight the journey to overcoming this challenge.

Identifying Triggers

Understanding what prompts procrastination is the first step toward overcoming it. Common triggers in dental school include:

- **Fear of Failure**: The pressure to excel can be daunting. Many students procrastinate because they fear their efforts won't meet expectations. This fear can lead to avoidance, creating a cycle of stress and anxiety.

- **Overwhelm**: The sheer volume of material to study can be intimidating. When faced with large projects or dense textbooks, it's easy to feel paralyzed and unsure of where to start.

- **Distractions**: Modern technology, particularly social media and mobile devices, can significantly disrupt focus. Notifications and the allure of scrolling can quickly eat into study time.

I vividly remember a semester when my procrastination led to a last-minute panic. I had an important exam approaching, and instead of starting my review weeks in advance, I found myself scrolling through social media and binge-watching series. The night before the exam, with hours of material to cover, I felt a surge of anxiety. It was a harsh wake-up call. I learned that recognizing my trigger—social media—was crucial. I decided to uninstall distracting apps during study hours, a decision that paid off immensely in subsequent semesters.

Strategies to Combat Procrastination

Now that we understand our triggers, it's time to implement strategies that can help mitigate procrastination.

Set Clear Goals

Breaking tasks into manageable parts and setting deadlines can dramatically improve focus and motivation. Here's how to do it effectively:

- **SMART Goals:** Specific, Measurable, Achievable, Relevant, and Time-bound goals help clarify what you want to achieve and create a sense of direction. For instance, instead of saying, "I'll study dental anatomy," you could set a goal: "I will study the muscles of mastication for one hour on Tuesday."

- **Daily and Weekly Goals:** Creating a daily to-do list or a weekly plan can provide structure to your study sessions. Each evening, I would outline what I aimed to accomplish the next day. This small habit kept me accountable and focused.

In my first semester, I set a goal to prepare for the semester exams by starting a study group. We would meet twice a week to discuss our topics, which kept everyone accountable. This collective effort not only motivated me but also reinforced my understanding of the material through teaching and discussion.

Reward Yourself

Introducing a reward system can be a powerful motivator. Here's how it can work:

- **Immediate Rewards:** After completing a study session or reaching a goal, allow yourself a small treat—like a favorite snack or a short episode of a show. This helps associate hard work with positive outcomes.

- **Long-Term Rewards:** Plan larger rewards for bigger achievements. For example, after finishing a difficult module, treat yourself to a weekend getaway or a dinner at your favorite restaurant. This can create a sense of anticipation and motivate you to complete tasks.

Creating a Productive Environment

Your study environment can significantly impact your ability to focus and get work done.

- **Designate a Study Space:** Having a dedicated area for studying, free from distractions, is crucial. This could be a specific desk at home or a quiet corner of the library.

- **Minimize Distractions:** Keep your study area organized and limit potential distractions. For instance, I transformed my cluttered desk into a serene workspace by organizing my materials and removing anything non-essential. This change positively affected my focus and productivity, allowing me to enter a more productive mindset when I sat down to study.

One particular moment stands out from my journey. I was preparing for a comprehensive practical exam that covered multiple subjects. Instead of studying gradually, I procrastinated, telling myself I had time. Days before the exam, I felt the weight of my choices—my stress was at an all-time high, and I realized I needed a serious change. I started using the Pomodoro Technique: studying for 25 minutes, followed by a 5-minute break. This method helped me maintain focus while providing structured breaks to recharge. Implementing these strategies not only improved my study habits but also helped me manage my anxiety effectively.

In conclusion, overcoming procrastination is a multi-faceted challenge, especially in the demanding environment of dental school. By identifying your triggers, setting clear goals, rewarding yourself, and creating a productive environment, you can develop a robust system to combat procrastination. Remember, it's about progress, not perfection, and every small step forward is a victory worth celebrating.

Chapter 7: Networking and Building Relationships

The Power of Connections

In the demanding journey of dental school, building strong connections is more than a luxury; it's essential for thriving. Relationships with mentors, faculty, and peers can provide the support, insight, and encouragement needed to navigate challenges and reach goals. Looking back, I realize that the connections I formed—from classmates who understood the stress of exams to mentors who shared wisdom beyond textbooks—were the foundation of my growth and resilience.

During my first semester, I met a senior student who profoundly shaped my journey. She could tell I was overwhelmed, trying to keep up with the fast-paced curriculum, and she went out of her way to help. She patiently explained concepts, shared study techniques, and showed me how to manage my time effectively. Her mentorship was not only an academic lifeline but also an emotional one, assuring me that I wasn't alone. Her guidance taught me that seeking help is a sign of strength and that we all need others to truly succeed.

The Importance of Mentors

Mentors bring a depth of understanding and perspective that textbooks simply cannot. They've experienced the pressures of dental school and can offer both professional guidance and personal encouragement. I found my first faculty mentor in Dr. Lee, a professor renowned for her expertise in restorative dentistry. Initially, I was intimidated to approach her, but one day after class, I took the leap and asked if she could help me understand a challenging topic. Her response was not only gracious but unexpectedly warm. She offered extra help and even shared stories of her own struggles as a student. Knowing that even accomplished professionals had once faced similar hurdles was a revelation, and it helped me feel capable of overcoming my own.

Dr. Lee's mentorship extended beyond academics; she encouraged me to attend seminars, introduced me to alumni, and provided advice on building my professional future. Her belief in me gave me the courage to explore research opportunities, which became a turning point in my academic career. That experience underscored the importance of mentors—sometimes, they see the potential in us that we have yet to recognize.

Building Relationships with Peers

While mentors guide us, peers walk alongside us, sharing the same challenges and victories. Building relationships with classmates creates a supportive environment where we can share resources, exchange ideas, and boost each other's morale. Early on, I was hesitant to join study groups, fearing I'd fall behind if others were ahead. But I quickly realized that study groups aren't about competing—they're about collaboration. In my first group, we not only helped each other with difficult material but also built friendships that made the stress of dental school feel lighter.

One memorable night, a group of us gathered to prepare for an anatomy exam, frantically reviewing diagrams and trying to memorize endless terminology. We were all exhausted, nerves fraying under the pressure. Suddenly, one of my friends made a joke that broke the tension, and soon we were all laughing. That moment of humor was a powerful reset. When we returned to studying, our focus had improved, and we tackled the material more effectively. I learned that sharing this journey with others can make the challenges feel smaller, reminding us that we're all in this together.

Tips for Networking and Asking for Help

Networking and asking for help can feel intimidating, especially when you're reaching out to people who seem like they have it all figured out. But here's a lesson I learned along the way: most people are happy to help if you approach them with sincerity and respect. Over time, I developed a few techniques that helped me form meaningful connections:

1. Start with Genuine Curiosity: When reaching out to someone, focus on asking questions that show genuine interest. Faculty members, alumni, or senior students have valuable experiences to share, and starting with thoughtful questions creates a natural way to connect. Rather than asking for favors right away, I found it helpful to start with, "What advice would you give a student in my position?"

2. Be Persistent but Respectful: Building connections takes time. If a faculty member doesn't respond to your first email or if a classmate doesn't immediately include you in a study group, don't be discouraged. I remember sending multiple emails to a professor before he was able to meet with me. He later told me that my polite persistence showed I was serious about learning. That experience taught me that persistence, paired with respect, is essential in forming connections.

3. Offer Help When You Can: Relationships are built on reciprocity. Even as students, we have something to offer, whether it's sharing resources, organizing study sessions, or simply being a supportive friend. During clinical rotations, I helped classmates who felt nervous about their first patient interactions. In return, they supported me through my own struggles, reinforcing the importance of mutual support.

4. Join Clubs or Study Groups: Professional and academic clubs are excellent for networking. I joined our school's dental student association, where I met students from different years who shared their insights and experiences. The association also hosted events with alumni and industry professionals, providing networking opportunities that would've been hard to find on my own.

Mentorship and Growth

One of my most transformative mentoring experiences came during an advanced clinical rotation. I was assigned to a senior dentist known for his high standards, and I was initially intimidated, unsure if I could meet his expectations. However, as I observed his meticulous approach to patient care, I learned more than just technical skills; I learned the importance of empathy and the art of building trust. One afternoon, he told me, "Patients may not remember everything you say, but they'll remember how you made them feel." That simple piece of advice stayed with me, shaping my approach to patient interactions. It was a powerful reminder that dentistry isn't just about procedures but about compassion and respect for each person in our care.

The Lifelong Value of Networking

In dentistry, the connections you make in school can continue to impact your career long after graduation. Peers who once sat beside you in lectures become colleagues and friends. Alumni who once struggled with the same challenges may later become mentors. I stay in touch with many friends I made in study groups, and we regularly check in on each other's progress. Recently, a classmate reached out to me with advice on a challenging case, sharing insights from his own practice that saved me hours of frustration.

Networking isn't about gaining something for yourself; it's about creating a professional community that values shared growth and mutual support. Relationships formed in dental school become the foundation of a strong, interconnected professional life.

In conclusion, cultivating relationships with mentors and peers is one of the most rewarding and essential aspects of dental school. Mentors provide wisdom and encouragement, while peers offer solidarity and camaraderie. Each connection, whether big or small, has the potential to shape your journey and make your time in dental school richer and more meaningful. Remember, networking isn't about attending formal events or making as many connections as possible. It's about building genuine relationships, offering support, and staying open to learning from those around you. The road through dental school can be challenging, but you don't have to travel it alone. By seeking out connections and being there for others, you'll find a world of support, knowledge, and friendship waiting for you.

Chapter 8: Building Self-Discipline in College Life

Self-discipline is more than a skill; it's the foundation that sustains your growth, helps you tackle challenges, and drives you toward your goals. In dental school, where the academic workload is demanding and time seems scarce, building self-discipline becomes essential for maintaining focus, completing tasks, and staying resilient. Here, we'll explore how creating routines, fostering accountability, staying motivated, and celebrating small achievements can not only improve your performance but make the journey through college life more manageable and fulfilling.

Establishing Routines: The Power of Consistency

Creating a structured daily schedule is one of the most effective ways to build self-discipline. A routine brings a sense of order and predictability that can help keep you grounded, even on days when motivation feels low or coursework is particularly challenging. Knowing exactly when and where to focus helps train your mind to shift into a productive state at the right times.

For me, establishing a morning routine was transform-ative. Initially, I found myself overwhelmed by the sheer number of tasks on my plate. Assignments, exams, and clinic hours piled up quickly. I decided to start small, committing to a simple morning ritual: I'd wake up, do a quick workout, have a balanced breakfast, and review my daily goals. This quiet time allowed me to mentally prepare for the day and reduced my stress levels. That commitment to a morning ritual set the tone for my day, giving me a steady foundation to tackle whatever challenges lay ahead.

To build your routine, think about what energizes and prepares you for the day. This could be anything from a brisk walk, meditation, or even a quick review of your lecture notes. Over time, routines become habits, freeing up mental space and helping you manage the unpredictable demands of college life.

Accountability: The Role of Study Buddies and Mentors

We often picture self-discipline as a solitary journey, but accountability can be a powerful motivator. Finding a study partner, joining a study group, or working with a mentor provides the encouragement needed to stay on track, even during the busiest times. A good study buddy not only makes study sessions more engaging but also creates a positive cycle of mutual support, where both of you benefit from the commitment to each other's progress.

During my second year, a close friend and I became study partners for our clinical theory exams. We'd set goals for each session and check in on each other's progress. On tough days, knowing I had to report my work kept me motivated. Our sessions became enriching discussions where we shared insights and resources, and knowing I had someone alongside me who understood my struggles was inspiring. That support proved invaluable when exam time arrived.

To build accountability, start small. Reach out to someone in your class who has similar study goals, or consider weekly check-ins with a mentor. Accountability doesn't just keep you disciplined—it also builds bonds and creates a shared sense of purpose.

Motivation Techniques: Staying Driven Through Visualization and Affirmations

Motivation is essential for self-discipline, but it can be fleeting, especially when the workload feels never-ending. To stay inspired, try using visualization and positive affirmations. Visualization involves picturing yourself achieving specific goals, like acing an exam or confidently handling patients in clinical rotations. Imagining these scenarios in vivid detail reinforces your commitment to putting in the work to reach those goals.

On days when I felt tempted to skip study sessions or cut corners, I would pause and imagine my future as a practicing dentist. I'd picture myself confidently interacting with patients, feeling fulfilled and capable in my role. This simple mental exercise reminded me that every small action I took contributed to that future reality.

Positive affirmations were equally powerful. I'd often remind myself, "I am capable, resilient, and moving closer to my goals every day." Repeating these affirmations countered self-doubt, giving me the strength to push through challenges. Find a few affirmations that resonate with your personal goals and use them as reminders on tough days.

Celebrating Small Wins: Recognizing Progress Along the Way

Self-discipline doesn't mean being relentlessly hard on yourself. Celebrating small accomplishments is essential for maintaining long-term motivation. Recognizing progress—whether it's finishing a difficult assignment or mastering a tough concept—reinforces your effort and reminds you of the strides you're making.

I remember a particularly challenging semester when I felt like I was barely keeping up. One evening, after completing a complex project, I decided to treat myself to my favorite dessert. That small act of self-care felt like a reward and renewed my energy. These little celebrations don't have to be grand—they can be as simple as acknowledging the work you've done and taking a well-deserved break.

Building in small rewards at the end of each week, like taking an afternoon off or watching a favorite show, reinforces your progress and keeps you energized. Reflecting on these wins also helps you stay positive and committed, even when the journey feels tough.

Personal Story: Discipline in Action

One of my most memorable experiences of discipline leading to success was during my third-year final exams. I had a series of exams back-to-back, and the stress was palpable. With deadlines looming, it would have been easy to let my routines slip and surrender to the chaos. But I knew that discipline was the only thing that would carry me through. I stuck to my daily study blocks, balanced with short breaks, and kept moments for exercise.

On the day of my last exam, I walked in feeling prepared and grounded. The discipline I'd cultivated throughout the semester helped me stay calm and collected, and as I finished my last exam, the sense of accomplishment was overwhelming. It wasn't just about the results; it was the realization that my dedication and consistency had enabled me to overcome one of the hardest weeks of my academic life.

The Bigger Picture: Why Self-Discipline Matters Beyond College

Self-discipline isn't just about surviving dental school; it's about building a foundation for your future career and personal growth. In dentistry—a profession where patients will rely on your expertise and dedication—the habits you build now will serve you throughout your life. The routines, accountability practices, and motivation techniques you adopt today will become the cornerstones of a successful, balanced career tomorrow.

Developing self-discipline takes effort, and it's normal to struggle along the way. But each small step strengthens your resolve and brings you closer to your goals. Remember, it's a journey—one that becomes easier with each stride. Celebrate your progress, stay committed, and know that every day you practice self-discipline, you're investing in a brighter, more resilient future.

Chapter 9: Maintaining Hygiene

The Importance of Personal Hygiene

In the world of dentistry, personal hygiene is not merely a routine; it is a fundamental commitment to excellence that reflects our dedication to oral health. As future dental professionals, we are charged with the responsibility of setting a standard—not only for ourselves but also for our patients. I remember vividly my first days in dental school, standing before the mirror, toothbrush in hand. Each stroke was not just about cleaning my teeth; it was about instilling confidence in myself and projecting professionalism. My morning rituals—brushing, flossing, and rinsing—became more than just self-care; they evolved into a commitment that I would carry into my practice.

The impact of good personal hygiene on our self-assurance cannot be overstated. I noticed a distinct difference in my engagement with peers and faculty when I felt fresh and clean compared to days when I let my routine slip due to the overwhelming pressures of exams or clinical work. One particular incident stands out during finals week when I hurried through my personal care, hoping to squeeze in a few extra minutes of study. That day, I felt less than my best during a crucial presentation, and my confidence wavered. It was a wake-up call that our profession demands more than technical skills; it requires a polished presentation, a strong personal ethic, and assurance in our capabilities, all deeply rooted in how we take care of ourselves.

Hygiene: A Student's Best Friend

Personal hygiene is paramount in dental school, not just for our patients but for our mental well-being as well. I learned this the hard way during a particularly stressful week when I allowed self-care to fall by the wayside. With back-to-back exams and looming project deadlines, I convinced myself that I simply didn't have time for personal care. Neglecting my hygiene routine left me feeling physically drained and mentally foggy, and it significantly affected my academic performance. That experience taught me that maintaining personal hygiene is not just an aspect of self-care; it is essential for sustaining both my health and academic success.

> **Tip:** Establish a hygiene routine that works for you. I found that even on my busiest days, dedicating just ten minutes to brush, floss, and rinse made a world of difference. I began to see my study area as an extension of myself, realizing that a clean study space was just as crucial as personal care. Decluttering my desk and organizing my materials not only created a more inviting atmosphere but also fostered a clear mind. A tidy environment promotes focus and clarity, which are essential for effective learning.

Reflecting on my experiences, I recognize the profound connection between personal care and academic success. When I walk into the clinic with my hair neatly tied back, a clean uniform, and fresh breath, I feel prepared. I am not just presenting myself as a future dentist; I am embodying the professionalism I aspire to project. Each time I interact with patients during clinicals, I am reminded that they deserve a practitioner who respects their own health and hygiene as much as they care for their patients' dental needs.

Keeping Your Study Space Clean

Our environment significantly influences our overall well-being. A clean study space not only enhances concentration but also boosts motivation. I discovered this during a hectic week when my study area became cluttered with notes, textbooks, and even empty coffee cups. I felt mentally bogged down and drained, leading to late-night cramming sessions and further neglect of my personal care. It wasn't until I took a few hours to organize my desk and clear away distractions that I noticed a significant change.

After cleaning, my productivity surged. I suddenly had space to breathe, think, and focus. I even added personal touches to my study area—a small plant and a few motivating quotes. These simple additions made my environment feel more inviting and enjoyable, reminding me that my hygiene practices encompassed more than physical cleanliness; they were also about nurturing my mental health.

The Role of Hygiene in Dental Practice

The connection between personal hygiene and professional practice cannot be overstated. In clinical settings, we represent not only ourselves but also our school and future profession. Patients expect a level of professionalism that begins with our appearance and extends to our practices. It is about more than just looking the part; it is about instilling confidence and trust in those we serve.

During my clinical rotations, I observed how maintaining a polished appearance could ease a patient's anxiety. On days when I felt particularly confident—dressed in a clean uniform with fresh breath and a smile—I noticed patients were more at ease. They engaged more openly, and their trust in my skills grew stronger. This relationship between appearance and patient comfort became an essential lesson in my training.

Personal Insight: Maintaining good hygiene serves as a foundation for professionalism and fosters respect and trust from those we serve. In dental practice, we are not merely treating teeth; we are caring for people who place their health in our hands. The impression we leave starts long before the first examination begins.

By prioritizing hygiene in our lives as dental students, we cultivate habits that will serve us and our patients well throughout our careers. The confidence that comes from presenting our best selves is invaluable, creating a ripple effect that enhances every interaction we have in this rewarding field. Embracing a routine of personal hygiene, combined with maintaining a clean study environment, not only enhances our professional image but also supports our mental well-being. Ultimately, it reinforces the belief that we are not just students; we are future healthcare providers, and that journey begins with how we care for ourselves.

Chapter 10: The Art of Staying Motivated and Managing Stress in Dental School

Navigating the demanding landscape of dental school can feel like an endless rollercoaster of exams, clinical rotations, and practical assessments. The pressure can be intense, especially during critical moments like final exams or mastering complex procedures in the clinic. It's easy to feel overwhelmed and lose motivation amid such challenges. However, fostering a resilient mindset can transform these struggles into opportunities for growth. In this chapter, I'll share insights on staying motivated and managing stress, enriched with personal anecdotes that illustrate these concepts.

Mindset Shifts: Reframing Struggles as Growth

One of the most powerful tools in maintaining motivation during tough times is the ability to reframe challenges as growth experiences. Instead of viewing an anatomy exam as a daunting hurdle, consider it an opportunity to deepen your understanding of the human body—an essential foundation for your future career.

During my second year, I faced a particularly gruelling practical exam in oral anatomy. As I entered the exam room, a wave of anxiety washed over me, coupled with self-doubt about my performance. But instead of succumbing to panic, I consciously shifted my perspective. I viewed the exam not merely as a test of my abilities, but as a chance to demonstrate my learning. This mental adjustment alleviated some of my anxiety and allowed me to engage more fully with the material.

One memorable moment during this process came during a comprehensive practical exam where we had to identify various anatomical structures on a model. Initially, I felt overwhelmed by the sheer volume of information. To cope, I created a mental map of the structures, connecting each one to its function and significance in dental practice. This visualization technique turned what felt like rote memorization into a meaningful learning experience, enriching my understanding and recall.

Managing Stress and Avoiding Burnout

The reality of dental school is that it can be incredibly demanding, often leading to stress and burnout. Balancing a packed schedule filled with lectures, clinical work, and personal commitments requires effective management strategies. It's essential to acknowledge the emotional toll this journey can take.

I remember a particularly challenging semester filled with back-to-back exams and clinical responsibilities. I felt stretched thin, battling waves of self-doubt and exhaustion. In this moment of struggle, I learned the importance of reaching out for support. Talking with my peers who were experiencing similar challenges not only alleviated my feelings of isolation but also provided a space for sharing strategies and coping mechanisms.

Mental Health Tips: To maintain balance during stressful periods, I discovered several effective techniques:

Exercise: Incorporating regular physical activity into my routine was a game changer. I took up running and found that it not only improved my physical health but also served as a mental reset. After a long day, a quick jog around the campus rejuvenated my spirit.

Mindfulness and Meditation: I began practicing mindfulness to stay grounded. Simple techniques, like focusing on my breath for a few minutes, helped calm my mind before high-stress situations, such as patient interactions or exams.

Nutrition: Paying attention to my diet made a notable difference in how I felt. I started preparing nutritious meals instead of relying on quick, unhealthy snacks, which significantly improved my energy levels.

Self-Care Practices: Prioritizing self-care is vital in the hectic life of a dental student. Schedule time for activities that recharge you. For example, I began reserving Sunday afternoons for self-care—whether it was going for a long run, indulging in a good book, or binge-watching my favourite series. This weekly ritual not only helped me unwind but also prepared me mentally for the upcoming week.

Building a Supportive Routine

Creating a daily routine that incorporates self-care and relaxation is essential for maintaining mental well-being. Designate specific times for study, exercise, and leisure activities. This structured approach can alleviate the chaos that often comes with a demanding academic schedule.

I vividly recall a week when I was overwhelmed with deadlines and clinical duties. In response, I created a detailed schedule that included blocks for study sessions, exercise, and even social time with friends. By adhering to this plan, I was able to regain control over my workload and mitigate feelings of burnout. My academic performance improved, and I felt more connected to my peers, reminding me of the importance of balance.

Staying motivated and managing stress are crucial components of thriving in dental school. By shifting your mindset to view challenges as opportunities for growth, prioritizing self-care, and fostering a supportive routine, you can navigate the demands of your education with resilience and confidence.

As you continue on this journey, embrace these techniques, adapt them to your personal style, and cultivate a mindset that sees challenges as stepping stones toward your future success. With determination and the right strategies in place, you'll emerge not only as a skilled dental professional but also as a well-rounded individual ready to make an impact in the field. Remember, it's not just about surviving dental school; it's about thriving and laying the groundwork for a successful career in dentistry.

Finding Balance in Dental School

Balancing the academic demands of dental school with personal life, friendships, and self-care is essential yet challenging. While the intensity of studies can make it tempting to devote all energy to coursework, sustaining that level of focus without taking time for yourself can quickly lead to burnout. Striking a balance isn't just about managing your time; it's about nurturing every aspect of your life so that you can approach each day with energy, resilience, and a clear mind. This chapter dives into the importance of balancing academics and personal life, making time for relaxation, fostering meaningful social connections, and embracing hobbies that bring joy.

Academic vs. Personal Life: Finding Harmony in the Juggle

Dental school demands an immense amount of focus, discipline, and time. Between lectures, clinical rotations, and exams, it can feel like there's hardly any room left for personal interests or a social life. Many students grapple with guilt when taking time away from studying, fearing it might hurt their performance. But in reality, prioritizing personal time can be essential—it lets you recharge, return to your studies with a fresh outlook, and ultimately perform better. Finding balance is about giving yourself permission to exist beyond the textbooks and clinical labs.

For me, this balance didn't come naturally; it was a conscious effort. Early in dental school, I was fully immersed in my studies, believing that the more time I devoted to coursework, the better I'd do. But I quickly found that spending every waking hour on academics wasn't sustainable. After feeling physically and mentally drained, I realized I needed to take control of my time. I began scheduling blocks of personal time—whether for exercise, cooking, or a quick walk in the park. This simple change gave me something to look forward to and provided mental clarity, making me more focused and effective in my studies.

To achieve this balance, acknowledge that personal time isn't a luxury but a necessity. Start by setting small, intentional breaks in your schedule, even if it's just 15 minutes for a coffee or a few minutes for a walk. Flexibility is key, but having a consistent routine can keep you grounded, especially when academic pressures start to peak.

Time for Yourself: Prioritizing Leisure for Mental Well-Being

Amid the whirlwind of exams and clinical work, it's easy to forget that relaxation is essential for mental and emotional health. Leisure activities allow your mind to rest, reducing stress and enhancing productivity. If you give yourself permission to unwind, you can actually avoid burnout and return to your studies with a fresher, more positive mindset.

When I began setting aside time for myself each week, I noticed a significant improvement in my mood and focus. I'd let myself get lost in a good novel for an hour or indulge in a comedy show on Netflix—a welcome escape from the academic world. One weekend, after a long and stressful week of exams, I spent an hour absorbed in a mystery novel. This small mental break felt like a reset. I realized that taking time to disconnect from my studies wasn't wasted time; it was an investment in my well-being. When I returned to my coursework, I felt clear-headed, more motivated, and ready to tackle complex topics with a renewed perspective.

To ensure you're giving yourself enough downtime, think about activities that genuinely make you feel relaxed. Whether it's listening to your favorite music, enjoying a warm cup of tea, or simply taking a walk in nature, let yourself enjoy this time without guilt. Know that these moments contribute significantly to your mental well-being and ultimately improve your academic performance.

Time for Hobbies: The Value of Pursuing Personal Interests

Hobbies are often the first things we set aside when academic demands intensify, yet they're an essential part of maintaining balance. Pursuing activities outside of schoolwork provides a much-needed creative outlet and joy, adding a sense of accomplishment beyond grades. Hobbies give us a space to express ourselves and often build resilience, offering something positive to return to when challenges arise.

For me, photography became a cherished hobby during dental school. On weekends, I'd grab my camera and explore local parks or neighbourhoods, capturing scenes that inspired me. I remember one particularly intense exam week. When the exams were finally over, I spent a Saturday morning photographing autumn leaves in the park. The colours, the crisp air, and the quiet time away from my studies allowed me to truly relax. When I returned to my coursework afterward, I was reinvigorated. Photography offered me both a mental escape and a source of happiness that grounded me through the toughest weeks.

To maintain balance, find a hobby that genuinely excites you and carve out time for it weekly. Whether it's sports, art, cooking, or playing an instrument, making space for something you love will add depth to your life. These activities aren't just "breaks" from studying; they're essential to building a well-rounded, fulfilling life.

Social Connections: The Importance of Building Supportive Relationships

While academics are crucial, so are the friendships and connections you build along the way. Forming meaningful relationships with classmates and peers can provide the emotional support and camaraderie that makes challenges more bearable. When surrounded by people who understand what you're going through, you gain strength and encouragement to navigate the rigorous demands of dental school. These friendships often provide perspective, helping you laugh when you feel overwhelmed and celebrate when you succeed.

One of my closest friendships in dental school started through a study group. We'd meet regularly, sometimes working late into the night, supporting each other through exams and assignments. One particular night, we were all exhausted, but we took breaks to chat about life outside of school, sharing funny stories and future goals. Those connections made the intense workload feel more manageable and created a sense of belonging. When exams were difficult or clinical work felt overwhelming, I knew I had friends who understood completely and could provide both empathy and motivation.

If you're struggling to find balance, reach out to classmates or join a study group. Make an effort to spend time with peers, even outside of academic settings. Social connections don't just support you academically; they add joy and companionship, lifting you up during challenging times and celebrating your successes along the way.

Finding Balance: A Lifelong Skill

Striking a balance between academics, personal interests, and social connections in dental school isn't easy, but it's a skill that will serve you for a lifetime. Each of these elements—time for yourself, hobbies, and relationships—plays a unique role in keeping you grounded, motivated, and resilient. Finding time for each part of your life creates a framework that supports both your academic success and personal well-being.

As you navigate dental school, remember that maintaining balance is essential not just for surviving these years but for thriving in your future career. Embrace this journey with an open mind and heart, recognizing that self-care, joy, and friendships are integral to long-term success. Life's greatest achievements aren't just about professional accomplishments but also about the relationships and memories we create along the way. So, cherish each moment, stay present, and know that finding balance is an ongoing journey—one that will enrich your life now and in the years to come.

Chapter 11: Laying the Foundation for Your Future in Dentistry

Preparing for a career in dentistry requires thoughtful planning, from identifying areas of interest to honing skills and developing lifelong learning habits. This chapter dives into setting early career goals, building a network, preparing for clinical practice, and navigating the transition from school to real-world dentistry.

Strategizing Your Specialization and Research Path in Dental School

One of the most valuable things you can do during dental school is to start thinking about potential specializations and research interests early. The field of dentistry offers a diverse range of paths, from orthodontics and oral surgery to periodontics and prosthodontics. Knowing where you might want to focus can make a significant difference in shaping your educational choices, extracurriculars, and ultimately, your career trajectory.

Start with Exploration

If you're leaning toward a particular branch, like oral surgery or orthodontics, it's essential to immerse yourself in these fields as soon as possible. Begin by exploring areas that naturally pique your curiosity within the core curriculum, elective classes, and hands-on training sessions. Make a list of specialties that seem exciting to you—maybe you've enjoyed a restorative dentistry rotation, or you found pathology especially intriguing. This list can serve as a guide for what you may want to dive deeper into.

Consider shadowing specialists whenever possible. Observing practitioners in a real-world setting will give you firsthand insight into the day-to-day challenges and rewards of different specialties. Some dental schools offer specialty-focused rotations or electives that allow you to experience aspects of multiple fields; make it a point to attend these if they're available.

Seek Out Mentors

Building a relationship with mentors is one of the most powerful steps you can take. Professors and clinicians are often more than willing to share their knowledge and can provide invaluable guidance on navigating your choices. Initiate conversations with professors whose lectures or seminars resonate with you. Ask for advice about the realities of a given specialty or for recommendations on how to strengthen your skills in a particular area. Remember, mentors can become advocates and provide networking connections that are invaluable in a competitive field.

One special tip: Try to attend as many specialty-focused seminars or workshops hosted by your school as you can. These events often feature experts discussing cutting-edge practices and advancements, allowing you to immerse yourself in the field's future. I remember attending a conference on digital orthodontics and realizing how transformative the field could be; it solidified my interest in the technical aspects of orthodontics and guided me to seek out further learning.

Engaging in Research Projects

For students with a research-oriented mindset, contributing to research projects can be one of the most enlightening experiences of your education. Look for ongoing projects at your institution and talk to faculty members about joining in any capacity, even if it's in a minor role such as data collection or literature review. This involvement can develop critical skills like data analysis and clinical reasoning, and also help you determine if a career in academia or research could be fulfilling for you.

From personal experience, reaching out to a professor about their research on minimally invasive surgical techniques transformed my outlook on dental procedures. The opportunity to assist with studies and learn about the intricacies of data collection showed me a whole new side of dentistry that goes beyond clinical practice. Research doesn't just look good on a resume—it builds your critical thinking and can deepen your interest in a specialty you hadn't previously considered.

Networking and Knowledge Building

In addition to your coursework, attending workshops, conferences, and even virtual seminars can broaden your perspective. Conferences are invaluable for connecting with both seasoned professionals and peers who share your interests. They also expose you to the latest research and technological advancements, which can be inspiring and motivating. Take time to ask questions, participate in discussions, and follow up with professionals you meet who might offer further insight or even mentorship.

Here's a special tip for making the most out of these events: come prepared with a list of questions or topics you're curious about. This shows initiative and helps you make a lasting impression on speakers or industry experts, who can become valuable connections down the road.

Tailoring Your Dental School Experience

Deciding on a specialization or committing to research is a journey. It doesn't all happen at once, and it's okay if your interests shift as you explore. By staying curious, proactive, and open to new experiences, you'll be better equipped to make an informed decision that aligns with your skills and aspirations. Above all, remember that your choices in dental school can lay the foundation for a rewarding, impactful career, so invest the time to learn about every opportunity and stay open to the paths you discover along the way.

Building a Network and Finding Mentors: Navigating Your Path in Dentistry

Mentorship is one of the most valuable assets you can have as a dental student. The guidance of an experienced mentor not only offers you a wealth of knowledge but also supports you through the unique challenges and rewards of the field. A good mentor can help you navigate clinical challenges, understand complex procedures, and even guide your career decisions. But finding the right mentor and building a strong network takes strategy, patience, and a proactive approach.

How to Identify and Connect with Mentors

The journey to finding a mentor often begins with those around you—professors, clinic supervisors, or even senior students and alumni. Start by identifying potential mentors who inspire you, either through their teaching style, area of expertise, or the way they approach patient care. Sometimes, the most approachable and understanding mentors are right in front of you in the classroom or clinic. Don't hesitate to introduce yourself after class, ask questions about their career path, or share your own aspirations.

Expressing genuine interest in their journey can open the door to a meaningful mentoring relationship.

Reaching out to alumni from your school who are now practicing dentists can be especially rewarding. Alumni often have a special connection to their alma mater and are generally open to sharing insights about their career paths, whether through formal alumni networks or informal conversations. When you connect with an alumnus, ask about their transition from student life to clinical practice, and inquire about any hurdles they faced and how they overcame them. Many professionals are not only willing to offer advice but enjoy the chance to give back to the next generation.

> **Special Tip:** Prepare a few thoughtful questions when reaching out to potential mentors, such as "What challenges did you face early in your career?" or "What do you think is the most important skill to develop as a dental student?" Being prepared shows respect for their time and makes the conversation more engaging for both of you.

The Power of Networking Events

Networking is a skill that pays off immensely, especially in a field as dynamic and interconnected as dentistry. Attending dental conventions, workshops, and seminars can broaden your perspective and introduce you to professionals from various specialties and backgrounds. Networking events are opportunities to not only gain knowledge but also make connections that can last throughout your career. Even if you feel a bit out of place at first, remember that everyone was once in your shoes. Push through the initial discomfort, and try to engage with people around you.

I remember attending my first networking event, feeling out of place among seasoned practitioners, but after a deep breath, I struck up a conversation with a dentist who later became a mentor and even helped me secure an internship. It was an opportunity that I would have missed if I had let my nerves hold me back.

Another fantastic way to meet people in the field is by joining dental associations and student organizations. Many of these groups host regular events, volunteer activities, and conferences where you can connect with like-minded peers and experienced practitioners. Volunteering for dental camps or awareness programs can give you a real-world perspective on public health, patient interaction, and team collaboration—all essential skills for a successful dental career.

Special Tip: Before attending networking events, do a bit of research on the speakers and attendees, if possible. A basic understanding of their work or achievements can help you initiate conversations and make a memorable impression.

Why Building a Network Matters

A strong network opens doors to internships, job opportunities, and collaborations. But beyond the professional benefits, it's also about building a support system in what can sometimes be a demanding and isolating career. A network of peers, mentors, and professionals creates a community that you can turn to for advice, motivation, and encouragement when times get tough.

At one conference, I spoke with a public health dentist who shared stories of working in underserved communities. That one conversation sparked a deeper interest in outreach and community health, opening up a new perspective on how I could use my career to make a meaningful difference.

Networking not only brings job prospects but can also broaden your vision of what dentistry can be.

Special Tip: Maintain connections by following up periodically. Send a quick email to update your mentors or networking contacts on your progress, thank them for their guidance, or share a resource they might find interesting. These small gestures keep the relationship strong and demonstrate your appreciation.

Mentorship and networking are invaluable in shaping your path in dentistry. Seek out mentors who resonate with you, and put yourself out there at events, even if it feels uncomfortable at first. These relationships will enrich your learning experience, provide career guidance, and connect you with a broader community of dental professionals. Remember, each interaction is an opportunity to learn something new and expand your possibilities. Whether it's a mentor who guides you through complex cases or a networking contact who inspires you with new ideas, the connections you make can be some of the most rewarding aspects of your career journey.

Staying Updated with Advancements and Building a Lifelong Learning Habit

Dentistry is one of the most dynamic fields, constantly shaped by technological advancements, innovative materials, and new approaches to patient care. Staying updated on these developments not only ensures that you remain competitive but also enhances the quality of care you provide. Building a habit of lifelong learning early in your career can make all the difference. I learned firsthand how committing to regular, structured learning allowed me to stay confident, relevant, and adaptable in practice.

Start Small: Incorporate Learning into Your Routine

One of the most effective ways to stay updated is by developing small, sustainable learning habits. Start by setting aside a bit of time each week to read articles, watch tutorials, or explore recent findings in dental journals. Rather than feeling pressured to read everything, pick a few reputable sources like the Journal of Dental Research or the British Dental Journal. Regular reading not only familiarizes you with advancements but also helps you understand current best practices that can be applied in your training.

If you're just starting, subscribing to a couple of newsletters from respected dental organizations can be a simple yet powerful way to stay in the loop. They often summarize recent research, highlight new technologies, and offer upcoming webinar opportunities. This way, even with a busy schedule, you get digestible updates without feeling overwhelmed.

Special Tip: Set a recurring reminder on your calendar for "Professional Reading" or "Dental Advances" once a week. This small commitment can make a huge difference over time and ensures learning doesn't get lost in a busy schedule.

Embrace Technology: Learn Today to Be Ready for Tomorrow

The rise of digital dentistry has already changed how we approach patient care. Technologies like CAD/CAM, 3D imaging, and digital X-rays are revolutionizing diagnostic capabilities and procedural accuracy. Familiarizing yourself with these tools during dental school prepares you for their integration in future practice. Not only will it give you an edge, but it will also help you become more comfortable with the digital aspects of patient care, which are rapidly becoming standard in the industry.

> **Special Tip:** Consider taking online courses or attending workshops specifically focused on new dental technologies. Platforms like Coursera and professional dental sites often offer affordable courses on CAD/CAM technology, 3D imaging, and digital diagnostics. Even if you aren't using these tools yet, understanding their applications gives you a solid foundation for future practice.

Lifelong Learning: Beyond Exams and Into Practice

Learning in dentistry shouldn't be solely exam-driven; it's a lifelong commitment. Building the habit of learning not just for exams, but for personal growth, helps you stay passionate and invested in the field. Make it a goal to learn something new each month, whether it's a clinical procedure, an updated treatment protocol, or a new way to enhance patient comfort.

Reflective practice can also enrich your learning journey. After attending a webinar, reading an article, or completing a practical, take a few moments to reflect on what you learned and how you might apply it. I've found that keeping a "learning journal" is especially helpful. After each significant learning experience, jotting down key takeaways, personal insights, and potential applications helps reinforce new information and gives you a record to look back on as you progress in your career.

Special Tip: Keep a digital or physical journal where you document these reflections. Not only will this help reinforce what you learn, but it will also be a valuable resource that you can revisit when you're working on cases that require particular skills or knowledge.

Engaging with the Dental Community

Dentistry, as much as it is a science, is also a community. Attending webinars, seminars, and conferences, even if only a few times a year, allows you to stay informed about industry shifts and interact with experts who offer different perspectives. At one conference I attended, I had the chance to listen to a panel on sustainable dental materials. The insights I gained influenced how I thought about material selection, and it opened my mind to the role of eco-friendly choices in dental practice. These events aren't just about learning; they're about connecting and being inspired by the broader goals of dentistry.

When attending these events, don't hesitate to engage with speakers or ask questions. These opportunities for direct learning are invaluable, and the discussions can provide deeper insight than reading alone. Additionally, participating in such events often provides continuing education (CE) credits, which are essential in most dental careers and contribute to your professional development.

Special Tip: After attending a conference or webinar, consider sharing what you've learned with your peers or colleagues. Teaching others reinforces your own understanding and can spark productive discussions on how to apply these new insights in practice.

Staying Inspired and Motivated

Finally, remember that lifelong learning is as much about personal motivation as it is about professional advancement. Keep reminding yourself why you chose dentistry and how staying updated helps you become the best version of yourself in your field. Learning doesn't have to feel like a chore. Keep things exciting by exploring topics that interest you personally—whether that's cosmetic dentistry, public health, or oral surgery.

In the end, staying updated isn't just about being competitive; it's about maintaining passion, staying inspired, and giving the best possible care to every patient you treat. With consistent effort, staying informed can become a fulfilling and integral part of your career journey.

Preparing for Real-World Practice: Transitioning from Student to Professional

The leap from dental school to professional practice marks one of the most profound transitions in your journey. In school, you grow comfortable in a structured environment, with guidance and feedback always within reach. However, stepping into the real world requires adaptability, resilience, and an ability to think on your feet. This journey is not solely about refining your technical skills—it's about developing the qualities that make you a trusted and capable dental professional. Here's a detailed roadmap on how to make the most of clinical training, learn from hands-on experiences, and prepare for the unique challenges and rewards of real-world practice.

From Classroom to Clinic: Navigating the Transition and Building Confidence

The shift from dental school to real-world practice can feel overwhelming as you leave behind the structured environment of the classroom for the dynamic, and sometimes unpredictable, world of clinical practice. Internships serve as a critical bridge, allowing you to observe how seasoned professionals handle diverse situations, manage patient expectations, and work collaboratively within a team. Internships are also your opportunity to experience firsthand the rhythm of a dental practice, from managing patient records to handling the pace of multiple patients in a day.

Every task is a learning opportunity, even the seemingly small ones. Assisting with procedures or managing patient flow provides insights into the daily operation of a dental practice. During my internship, I kept a small notebook to jot down observations, questions, and techniques. One of the best pieces of advice I received early on was to treat every day as a learning experience. Don't hesitate to ask questions—most experienced dentists remember their early days and are often more than happy to offer tips and stories to help you along.

Special Tip: Make a checklist of essential soft skills—such as patient communication, time management, and teamwork. Set a personal goal to improve one skill each week. Focusing on these areas during your internship not only builds your confidence but also gives you valuable insights into the realities of practice.

The Human Element: Learning to Connect with Patients

In real-world practice, dentistry is as much about understanding people as it is about clinical technique. Every patient you encounter brings their own personality, concerns, and expectations. Learning to connect with them on a personal level is key to gaining their trust. While school provides the technical foundation, real-world practice teaches you the importance of compassion and communication in patient care.

Reflecting on my own experience, I recall one of my first interactions with an extremely anxious patient. Despite feeling confident in my technical skills, I quickly realized that her anxiety required a new approach. I took a few extra moments to explain each step, ensuring she felt informed and at ease. Experiences like this taught me that dentistry isn't just about procedures—it's about building trust, easing fears, and showing empathy. These soft skills may not be part of your curriculum, but they are integral to becoming a respected dental professional.

Special Tip: Practice active listening. Small gestures, like reflecting a patient's concerns or explaining procedures in layman's terms, make a big difference. Simple phrases like, "I understand you're feeling anxious about this" or "I'm here to help you feel comfortable" reassure patients, build trust, and improve the overall experience.

Overcoming Challenges: Building Resilience in Real-World Dentistry

In the real world, dentistry requires quick thinking, flexibility, and composure in the face of challenges. Time management becomes essential as you juggle appointments, manage unforeseen delays, and work to stay efficient without compromising patient care. Unlike school, where procedures are taught in a step-by-step, controlled manner, real-world dentistry often demands on-the-spot decision-making and adaptability.

Early in my practice, I faced a complex case involving a patient with multiple oral health issues and limited time. I had to make swift, informed decisions to prioritize treatments, which taught me that being a professional isn't about knowing everything; it's about remaining composed, resourceful, and knowing when to seek guidance or refer to a specialist. Experiences like these build resilience, helping you grow comfortable with the unpredictable nature of dentistry.

Special Tip: Develop a mental toolkit of problem-solving strategies. When faced with a challenging case, take a moment to pause, assess, and consider your options. Don't hesitate to consult with colleagues or mentors for advice. This skill builds confidence and prepares you to handle complex cases with a steady approach.

Preparing for the Reality of Practice Management

If you're planning to run your own practice, understanding the operational side of dentistry is essential. Internships and early job experiences are invaluable for this, providing insights into patient flow, coordination among team members, and administrative responsibilities. Learning these practical skills—like managing schedules, understanding billing, and coordinating with staff—sets you up for success when you eventually take on the responsibility of practice ownership.

During my internship, I took time to observe how patient records were managed, shadowed the office manager, and learned about appointment scheduling to minimize wait times. Understanding these details goes beyond clinical skills; it prepares you for the complete patient experience that defines a well-run practice.

> **Special Tip:** If you're serious about owning a practice, consider taking a basic business course or reading about practice management. Gaining a foundational understanding of business principles will make the transition smoother and allow you to focus on providing excellent patient care while managing a successful practice.

Building Confidence Through Practice and Peer Learning

Mastering clinical skills requires consistent practice, especially outside class hours. Set aside extra time to practice in the simulation lab, focusing on techniques that require muscle memory and precision. The more familiar you become with procedures, the more confident you'll feel in real patient interactions.

Peer learning is equally valuable. Collaborating with classmates creates an environment where everyone benefits from shared insights, techniques, and feedback. In my own training, study groups often revealed small but impactful techniques I hadn't considered. A friend once showed me an alternative approach to matrix placement in restorations that made my work significantly easier. Peer support builds not only clinical knowledge but also emotional resilience—a valuable asset in the sometimes stressful environment of clinical practice.

Special Tip: Form a study group for clinical sessions, where you can watch, provide feedback, and practice procedures together. These shared experiences foster an invaluable support network that not only builds your skills but also provides emotional encouragement.

Embracing a Lifelong Learning Mindset

Transitioning from student to professional is a journey of continual growth. In real-world practice, each patient encounter, each challenge, and each success contributes to your development. Embrace each experience, learn from mistakes, and reflect on your progress. Over time, you'll find that these moments—however challenging—are shaping you into a more skilled and compassionate professional.

Resilience, humility, and a commitment to growth are the cornerstones of a successful dental career. As you gain experience, you'll discover that dentistry is about making a difference, one patient at a time. The skills, insights, and relationships you build now will form the foundation of a career that is both rewarding and impactful.

Special Tip: Keep a "practice log" where you jot down your reflections after each day. Note what went well, what you found challenging, and areas for improvement. This habit not only helps you track your growth but also serves as a reminder of how far you've come.

By embracing hands-on practice, learning from peers, and reflecting on personal experiences, you'll be well-equipped to transition smoothly from student to professional. This journey is one of self-discovery, where each experience builds your technical competence, confidence, and compassion. Remember that every challenge you face brings you one step closer to becoming a skilled, thoughtful, and resilient dental professional.

Embracing Growth and Resilience on the Path to Professionalism

The journey from dental school to clinical practice is a challenging but profoundly rewarding path, one that transforms you from a student into a skilled, compassionate, and adaptable professional. Each step—from finding mentors to mastering hands-on techniques—brings valuable experiences that go beyond textbooks and exams, shaping both your technical skills and your character. The ups and downs you encounter along the way teach resilience, humility, and a deeper understanding of the human aspect of patient care.

Preparing for a career in dentistry isn't just about acquiring knowledge; it's a personal evolution. Each lesson you learn now, whether from a challenging case, a patient interaction, or a supportive mentor, helps you grow into a confident and capable practitioner. The skills you're developing have the power to make a lasting impact on patients' lives, so embrace each lesson, continually seek knowledge, and view every experience as an opportunity for growth.

As you navigate your career, planning for the future and preparing for clinical practice are integral milestones. Embrace every chance to learn, actively seek mentors, and engage with the dental community. Each experience—whether it's a complex case, a collaborative peer learning session, or an insightful conversation with a mentor—shapes not only your clinical skills but also enriches your perspective on the field and your role within it.

The transition from the structured environment of school to the unpredictable reality of practice can feel daunting. But remember, each challenge you face is an invaluable learning experience. Approaching this journey with an open mind will help you develop the resilience needed to handle real-life situations. Lean on your peers and mentors for support and guidance; together, you'll navigate the intricacies of dentistry, building the confidence, patience, and skill essential to thriving in the profession.

Real-world practice is a continuous process of learning, adapting, and self-discovery. Every patient interaction, every procedure, and even every mistake contributes to your growth as a clinician. These moments teach you that dentistry is not just about technical skill—it's about empathy, adaptability, and resilience. With each case, you'll refine your techniques, learn to communicate with compassion, and gain the confidence to handle unexpected challenges.

Preparing for practice means equipping yourself not only with technical abilities but also with a mindset geared toward lifelong learning and personal development. Great practitioners don't just treat teeth; they connect with their patients, understand their concerns, and adapt to their unique needs. Embrace each challenge as it comes, knowing that it's a stepping stone toward becoming a skilled, compassionate, and resilient dental professional.

The Conclusion

Embracing the Journey

As you stand at the threshold of your dental career, it's essential to take a moment to pause and reflect on the path that has brought you here and the road that lies ahead. The journey through dental school is not merely a series of exams and clinical hours; it's a transformative experience that shapes not only your professional skills but also your character and resilience. Each lecture, every late-night study session, and each interaction with patients has been a step towards your goal of becoming a compassionate, skilled dentist.

Reflection: Celebrating Your Progress

Now is the time to celebrate how far you've come. Reflect on the challenges you've faced and the growth that has stemmed from them. Think back to the late nights spent poring over textbooks, the exhilaration of mastering a new skill in the clinic, and the satisfaction of helping a patient find relief from pain. Each of these moments represents a significant milestone on your journey, building your confidence and competence.

Take a moment to appreciate those small victories— whether it's acing a tough exam, successfully performing a procedure for the first time, or simply deepening your understanding of a complex topic. These moments, no matter how minor they may seem, are the stepping stones that propel you forward and remind you of your passion for dentistry.

Special Tip: Create a "Success Journal" where you record your achievements, no matter how small. Reviewing your accomplishments can boost your morale during challenging times and provide tangible evidence of your progress.

This reflection is more than just looking back; it's about recognizing the lessons learned and the resilience developed along the way. Ask yourself: What have these experiences taught you about yourself? How have you adapted to the pressures and demands of dental school? Acknowledging your growth reinforces your ability to overcome obstacles and prepares you for the challenges that lie ahead.

The Impact of Your Work on Patients

As you prepare to transition from student to professional, keep in mind the profound impact your work will have on your future patients. Dentistry is not merely about fixing teeth; it's about improving lives. You have the power to restore confidence through a healthy smile, provide comfort to someone in pain, and educate individuals about the importance of oral health. Your commitment to learning and growing in this field will shape the experiences of those who rely on you for care.

Always remember that each patient is a unique individual, bringing their own stories, challenges, and hopes into your chair. Embracing this perspective will enrich your practice and help you connect with your patients on a deeper level. The work you do will extend beyond the dental chair, making a real difference in their lives and fostering lasting relationships built on trust and understanding.

Special Tip: Develop a patient-centered approach by actively listening to your patients' concerns and tailoring your communication to their needs. Building rapport not only improves patient satisfaction but also enhances the effectiveness of your treatments.

Final Thoughts: Embracing Challenges as Opportunities

As you continue your journey, remind yourself that every challenge is an opportunity for growth and learning. The road through dental school is designed to push your limits, and it is within these moments of discomfort that you will discover your true potential. Embrace the setbacks as integral parts of your learning journey. They will teach you resilience, problem-solving skills, and the importance of seeking help when needed.

Surround yourself with a supportive network of peers, mentors, and faculty. Don't hesitate to lean on them during tough times; they understand the struggles you face and can offer guidance and encouragement. Share your experiences, collaborate on difficult subjects, and support one another in both academic and personal endeavors. This camaraderie will not only ease the journey but will also enrich it, allowing you to learn from one another's experiences.

Special Tip: Regularly attend networking events, workshops, and seminars to expand your professional network. Building strong relationships with mentors and peers can provide invaluable support and open doors to future opportunities.

Final Words of Advice for Dental Students

As you embark on this exciting chapter, carry with you these key pieces of advice:

Resilience: The ability to bounce back from setbacks is crucial. Don't be discouraged by failures; instead, view them as lessons that will ultimately make you a better dentist. Every stumble is a chance to grow stronger.

Passion: Let your love for dentistry shine through in everything you do. This passion will be your greatest motivator, inspiring you to keep learning and growing, even when the going gets tough.

Support Network: Surround yourself with individuals who uplift and inspire you—whether they are peers, mentors, or family. This network will be invaluable as you navigate the complexities of dental school and beyond.

Remember, this journey is uniquely yours. Embrace each moment, cherish your experiences, and always keep your ultimate goal in sight: to become a compassionate, skilled, and dedicated dentist who makes a difference in the lives of your patients. Each day you invest in your education is a step toward realizing that goal, and every challenge you face will only serve to strengthen your resolve. You are not just studying for exams; you are preparing to transform lives.

So, move forward with confidence, curiosity, and a commitment to make your mark in the world of dentistry. The road ahead may not always be smooth, but it is undoubtedly worth it. Your dedication to this profession will shape not only your career but also the lives of many—making every effort you invest today a valuable contribution to a brighter tomorrow. Embrace the journey, learn from every experience, and never lose sight of the impact you can make.

As you step into your professional life, carry the lessons of resilience, empathy, and continuous learning with you. These qualities will not only make you a successful dentist but also a trusted and beloved member of your community. Your journey has equipped you with the tools to face any challenge, the knowledge to provide exceptional care, and the heart to make a meaningful difference in the lives of your patients.

Congratulations on reaching this pivotal moment. The future of dentistry is in your hands, and with your passion and dedication, it's sure to be bright.

Final Tip: Continue to seek out opportunities for professional development even after graduation. Whether it's pursuing further specialization, attending advanced workshops, or contributing to dental research, staying engaged in lifelong learning ensures that you remain at the forefront of your field, ready to offer the best care to your patients.

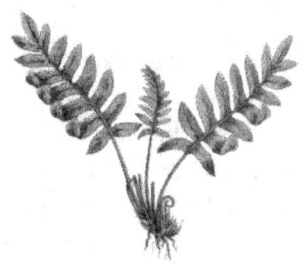

Fern,

Because it symbolises adaptability and resilience in the face of ever changing world

Acknowledgements

As I reach the conclusion of this journey, I want to express my heartfelt gratitude to those who have played an instrumental role in my development as both a dental student and an individual.

First and foremost, I extend my deepest appreciation to my mentors and faculty members. Your guidance, wisdom, and dedication to teaching have shaped my understanding of dentistry and inspired my passion for this profession. Thank you for your insightful feedback and for fostering an environment that encouraged curiosity and growth. Your commitment to student success is truly admirable and has made a significant impact on my educational journey.

To my peers and classmates, I am grateful for the camaraderie and shared experiences that made this challenging journey more enjoyable. Together, we've celebrated victories, navigated challenges, and created memories that I will cherish for a lifetime. Your support and collaboration have enriched my learning experience and have made me a better student and future dentist.

I wish to thank my family, whose unwavering encouragement and belief in my abilities have been my greatest source of strength. Their patience during the late nights and long study sessions kept me motivated, and their love has been a constant reminder of why I embarked on this path in the first place.

I also want to acknowledge the countless patients who have allowed me to learn from them during my clinical experiences. Your trust in me during my education has reinforced my commitment to providing compassionate care and understanding the importance of the dentist-patient relationship. You are the reason I strive to become the best dentist I can be.

Lastly, a special thanks to all the authors, researchers, and practitioners whose work has informed and inspired this book. Your contributions to the field of dentistry have paved the way for future generations and continue to shape the landscape of oral health care.

As I move forward in my dental career, I carry with me the lessons learned and the relationships built during this journey. Thank you all for being part of this experience. Your influence has been invaluable, and I am excited to embrace the future with all of you in mind.

About the Author

Dr. M. Azar is a dedicated dentist and passionate advocate for dental education, combining clinical expertise with a commitment to the well-being of future dental professionals. Having navigated the rigorous journey of dental school and transitioned into practice, Dr. M. Azar understands the unique challenges and triumphs that define a dental student's path. This background fuels their drive to support students in excelling academically, developing resilience, and fostering a balanced life, all while maintaining a commitment to compassionate patient care.

Graduating from P. M . Nadagouda Memorial Dental College and Hospital, Bagalkot, India, Dr. M. Azar has gained a deep appreciation for the complexities of dentistry—not only as a science but as an art that touches lives. Recognizing that success in this field requires more than technical skill, Dr. M. Azar approaches dentistry with empathy and a focus on building trusting, supportive relationships with patients. This perspective shapes their practice, emphasizing patient comfort, understanding, and a collaborative approach to health care.

In addition to their work in clinical dentistry, Dr. M. Azar is an advocate for mental health and self-care in the dental community. Drawing on personal experiences and lessons learned from mentors, they are committed to helping dental students and new practitioners build strong foundations for their careers. Dr. M. Azar is actively involved in mentoring, offering guidance through workshops and writing, and sharing effective study techniques, time management strategies, and self-care practices that foster well-rounded growth. They believe that a thriving dental professional balances the demands of the profession with personal well-being and resilience, setting an example for others in the field.

Outside of their practice and educational pursuits, Dr. M. Azar finds joy in philately, gardening, and a variety of other activities, whether it's exploring nature, delving into new advancements in dental technology, or spending quality time with loved ones. These interests provide balance and fresh perspectives, helping to cultivate creativity and inspiration that inform their approach to dentistry.

Through this book and their ongoing mentorship, Dr. M. Azar aims to empower the next generation of dental professionals to embrace both the challenges and rewards of their journey. Their message is one of resilience, compassion, and continuous growth, encouraging students to approach their studies and careers with confidence, curiosity, and a steadfast commitment to making a difference in the lives of their patients.

ISBN-13: 9781234567890
ISBN-10: 1477123456

Cover design by: Art Painter
Library of Congress Control Number: 2018675309
Printed in the United States of America